HYPERTENSION
AND YOU

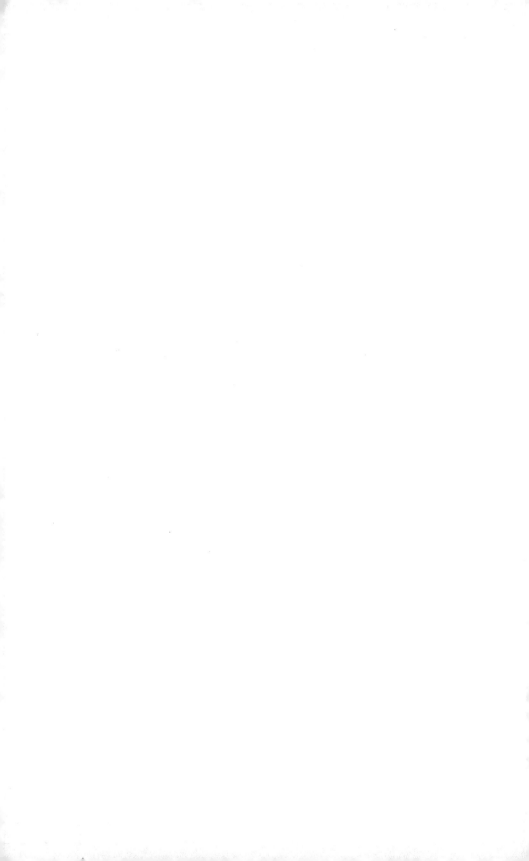

HYPERTENSION AND YOU

Old Drugs, New Drugs, and the Right Drugs for Your High Blood Pressure

Samuel J. Mann, MD

ROWMAN & LITTLEFIELD PUBLISHERS, INC.

Lanham • Boulder • New York • Toronto • Plymouth, UK

Published by Rowman & Littlefield Publishers, Inc.
A wholly owned subsidiary of The Rowman & Littlefield Publishing Group, Inc.
4501 Forbes Boulevard, Suite 200, Lanham, Maryland 20706
www.rowman.com

10 Thornbury Road, Plymouth PL6 7PP, United Kingdom

British Library Cataloguing in Publication Information Available

Library of Congress Cataloging-in-Publication Data
Mann, Samuel J., 1948-
  Hypertension and you : old drugs, new drugs, and the right drugs for your high blood pressure / Samuel J. Mann.
     p. cm.
     ISBN 978-1-4422-1517-7 (pbk. : alk. paper)—ISBN 978-1-4422-1519-1 (electronic)
     1. Hypertension—Popular works. 2. Hypertension—Chemotherapy. 3. Self-care, Health—Popular works. I. Title.
  RC685.H8M284 2012
  616.1'32061—dc23   2012004618

∞™ The paper used in this publication meets the minimum requirements of American National Standard for Information Sciences—Permanence of Paper for Printed Library Materials, ANSI/NISO Z39.48-1992.

Printed in the United States of America

CONTENTS

LIST OF ABBREVIATIONS

Throughout the book, I will use some convenient abbreviations that are widely used in the medical literature. They are listed below for easy reference.

Hypertensive mechanisms:

RAS   renin-angiotensin system
SNS   sympathetic nervous system

Drug classes:

ARB   angiotensin receptor blocker
ACEI   angiotensin-converting enzyme inhibitor
CCB   calcium channel blocker
DRI   direct renin inhibitor

Drugs:

HCTZ   hydrochlorothiazide

INTRODUCTION

Although John takes three drugs for his hypertension, his blood pressure is still 150/100, and he remains at increased risk of stroke or heart attack. *Comment: John does not have uncontrollable hypertension. He is on the wrong drugs.*

Sarah's blood pressure is a perfect 120/80 on two drugs. But she feels tired. *Comment: Sarah feels tired because she is on the wrong drugs.*

Bill is taking four antihypertensive drugs, and his blood pressure is well controlled. But the drugs are costing him $3,000 a year. *Comment: Bill is probably on more drugs than he needs, and is on more expensive drugs than he needs, because he is on the wrong drugs.*

Seventy-five million Americans have hypertension. Whether they like it or not, most will end up requiring medication. **If you have hypertension and are on medication, how well your blood pressure is controlled, how you feel, and how long you will live all depend on whether you are on the medication that is right for you.**

Unfortunately, **there is something terribly wrong with the current drug treatment of hypertension.** Over 35 percent of people taking blood pressure medication still have elevated readings.[1] Millions are living with avoidable side effects, are on more drugs than they need, are paying too much, or are taking medication even though they don't really need it.

Millions wrongly believe either that their blood pressure cannot be controlled or that lifelong side effects are the "cost" of having a normal blood pressure.

In many instances, doctors, despite good intentions, are not prescribing the medications, dosage, or combinations that are best suited for their patients, unaware there are better ways to prescribe. This is a very widespread problem, and it is fixable.

This book is about the drug treatment of hypertension. It is about what is wrong with how blood pressure medications are prescribed and about how to get it right to maximize blood pressure control, minimize side effects, and reduce the amount and cost of your medication.

HOW THIS BOOK DIFFERS FROM OTHER BOOKS ON HYPERTENSION

Most books on hypertension focus on what readers can do to avoid medication. There is no question that sustained lifestyle changes can reduce and in some cases even eliminate the need for medication, and are extremely beneficial to health in many important ways. I don't focus on lifestyle changes in this book, not because they aren't important but because I have little to add that hasn't already been written. Also, whether they like it or not, of the 75 million people with hypertension, about 50 million have ended up on medication.[1] I am writing this book for that 50 million, many of whom can do better than they are doing.

Hypertension and You focuses on the blood pressure medications. Unlike other books, it doesn't just rehash the usual standard information, such as the dosage range and lists of side effects. It conveys what is not discussed in other books, focusing on whether or not you are on the drugs, dosage, and combinations that are right for you and most likely to control *your* hypertension without side effects. It can lead to changes in your treatment and outcome.

Other books that discuss blood pressure medications don't convey the problems with how they are prescribed or that different people do better with different drugs. They pay inadequate attention to old and forgotten drugs that can control hypertension at a lower cost than the newest drugs. They don't reveal which of the new drugs are worth the cost and which are not.

I will identify those drugs. I will name the biggest offenders in terms of side effects and the drugs to consider instead of them. I will describe better ways of using the medications you are familiar with, and will introduce you to wonderful, but woefully underused, medications you and even your doctor might not be familiar with.

I will also focus on drug combinations. Half of people taking medication for hypertension require more than one drug and depend on their doctor to prescribe the right combination and dosage. However, ineffective combinations are often prescribed, resulting in inadequately controlled hypertension requiring yet more drugs, in unnecessary side effects, and in unneeded costs. I will present logical strategies that can be helpful in selecting and combining drugs. I will present information that you can bring to your doctor, who then can make changes to your treatment that can help control your blood pressure with fewer drugs, without side effects, and with lower costs.

I will emphasize, more than any previous books do, **the importance of finding the right fit, finding the medication and the dosage that is right for *you*.** I will describe the clues that can help identify the drugs that are most likely to lower *your* blood pressure, and those that are least likely to lower it. Even an excellent drug can be the wrong drug for *you*.

THE IMPORTANCE OF THE RIGHT MEDICATION

The great news is that we have many effective drugs that lower blood pressure, prevent heart attacks and strokes, and, if prescribed wisely, can bring hypertension under control in almost everyone with hypertension. They are lengthening the lives of millions. That's why I am an unconflicted advocate for prescribing antihypertensive medications in people who need them.

The bad news though is that **the treatment of hypertension is nowhere near as good as it could be**. Week after week, as a hypertension specialist, I see new patients who don't feel well on their medication or whose blood pressure is uncontrolled on three or more medications. For most, all that is needed is adjustment of the medication. **What we need, in terms of medication, is already out there. We just need to use it better**.

Nearly every drug, *on average*, lowers blood pressure by about as much as any other drug. But in most individuals, certain drugs lower blood pressure much more than others do. The drug that is right for you will lower your blood pressure; the wrong drug won't. That is why getting onto the right drug is the key to controlling your hypertension with the fewest medications possible.

Millions of people who are taking their medication regularly aren't getting the results they should be getting. If you are going

to be taking blood pressure medication for the rest of your life, it is imperative to get it right. Often, all that is needed is a little tweaking of the medication. Unfortunately, for millions, that tweaking never gets done. **Ironically, in this age of soaring medical costs, getting it right would not increase drug costs.** It would actually reduce them, while also preventing more strokes and heart attacks.

We can and must make better use of the medications available today because, frankly, there are no new breakthrough drugs on the horizon. Over the past few decades, one new drug after another has entered the market. That era is over. With all the medications available today, there is little likelihood that any new drug can become a blockbuster. So it makes little sense for the pharmaceutical industry to invest the half billion dollars needed to develop a new drug and perform the trials needed for FDA approval. They have moved on to other pastures. Fortunately, we already have the drugs that can do the job. We don't need new drugs. We just need to make better use of the drugs we have.

What I will convey is not theoretical; it reflects what I do with patient after patient, day after day. I will provide you with information that you can discuss with your physician to help achieve better blood pressure control with fewer side effects and, very possibly, with less medication. I will convey information that your doctor probably has not told you, some of which he might not even know.

MY VIEW AS A HYPERTENSION SPECIALIST

When I started out in medicine, I saw many patients whose lives had been devastated by a stroke caused by hypertension. Only in their sixties or seventies, they would arrive in a wheelchair, their left or right side paralyzed. Some could speak normally; some couldn't. I always considered a stroke one of the worst things that could happen because of the suddenness and, in many cases, the irreversibility.

The statistics tell us that in this era of hypertension treatment, we have reduced the incidence of stroke by 40 percent. I believe that statistic, but I also believe it greatly understates the potential of hypertension treatment. I was chatting with my colleagues at the Hypertension Center, and, even though almost all of our patients have hypertension, none of us could remember the last time we had seen a patient with controlled hypertension who had suffered that classic devastating stroke. Yes, we had patients well into their eighties who suffered small strokes due to disease in small arteries that accompanies advanced aging. Yes, we had patients who had strokes caused by other reasons, such as propagation of a clot from the heart. But we had not been seeing, in our well-controlled hypertensive patients, any of the devastating hypertensive strokes we used to see.

I don't mean to suggest that successful treatment of hypertension can prevent 100 percent of strokes. If we live long enough, of course we can suffer a stroke. And diabetes, smoking, elevated cholesterol levels, and genetic predisposition increase the risk of stroke even in people with well-controlled hypertension or no hypertension. But my experience, and that of my colleagues, suggests that we can prevent substantially more than 40 percent of major strokes, maybe 80 or 90 percent. This would not be a result of treating hypertension; it would be a result of successfully treating hypertension, meaning getting the blood pressure down to normal.

WHY ARE SO MANY PEOPLE GETTING THE WRONG MEDICATION?

If we have so many good medications, why is hypertension uncontrolled in so many Americans, and why are so many patients suffering side effects? In many cases, it is because patients are not taking their medications regularly. But in many others, it is because patients who are taking their medication regularly are on the wrong medication. Different people need different medications and different doses and different combinations, and they are not getting the medication, dose, or combination that is right for them.

There are many reasons why. First, the devil is in the details, and most doctors don't have the intimate knowledge of the many blood pressure medications that is needed to prescribe them in the best way. General practitioners and internists are not specialists or experts in treating hypertension, nor are most nephrologists and cardiologists. As is the case with many other medical conditions, there are now so many medications to choose from that many generalists do not know enough of the intricacies and nuances to make the best use of them. And prescribing the same medication to patient after patient just does not cut it.

Getting the job done right is about the details—the details of your hypertension and the details of the drugs being used. These are the details I will be discussing in this book.

If you have mild, easy-to-control hypertension, your doctor can throw almost any medication at you, with a 40 percent or so chance of normalizing your blood pressure with the first drug he prescribes. If this is the case, and you are taking one medication and your blood pressure is normal and you feel great, you probably don't need to read this book. However, if your hypertension is more severe or hasn't been brought down to truly normal by the first drug or two, your doctor might be unclear as to what to do next. He might simply add drugs without any clear strategy, hoping your blood pressure will fall. There are a great many nuances in selecting and combining blood pressure medications.

Another problem is the huge role of marketing. With great marketing, a mediocre drug can become the number-one seller. With poor marketing, a great drug never makes it and is ultimately forgotten. The newest, most expensive medications are promoted aggressively. Some are terrific drugs; some aren't. Meanwhile, some terrific and inexpensive older drugs are no longer promoted, and many doctors, unaware of them, rarely prescribe them. Worse, some are no longer available; because of their diminishing sales, they are not profitable, and no one produces them anymore.

Finally, the published medical research that doctors rely on focuses mostly on the newer, expensive drugs. Studies focus on showing that the drugs, on average, lower blood pressure, rather than on identifying who is likely to respond to their drug and who is not. A pharmaceutical corporation is not interested in identifying the 20 or 30 percent of people most likely to respond to their drug. They want everyone on their drug.

YOU AND YOUR DOCTOR

Where will the information in this book fit with regard to your relationship with your doctor? Certainly I am not recommending that you treat your own hypertension, or change medication or dosage on your own. What I hope to do is to communicate that **if your blood pressure is not controlled, if you are living with side effects, if you believe you are on too much medication, or are paying too much, you are probably not on the right medications, and there are excellent alternatives you should know about.** It is my aim to supply you with information and alternatives that you can discuss with your physician, with the goal of improving the drug therapy of your hypertension. I hope many internists and other physicians will also read this book, since I will be conveying information that will be informative to them as well.

WHY NOT NONDRUG THERAPY?

As a specialist in hypertension, I have treated many patients who prefer to avoid medication, both because they don't like taking medication and because of concern about side effects. I support their effort to adopt healthy habits, and there is no doubt that a healthy lifestyle, in particular a healthy diet, weight loss, reduction of sodium intake, and exercise, can lower blood pressure and reduce, and, in some, eliminate, the need for medication. There is no doubt that losing 30 pounds and keeping them off can have a sizeable effect on your blood pressure and your health in general.

However, the effects of lifestyle changes in the management of hypertension are not unlimited. Blood pressure readings may drop, but in many, particularly those with more than mild hypertension, not enough. Even with a healthy lifestyle, many will still need medication to bring their blood pressure down to truly normal. But clearly, even if a healthy lifestyle doesn't normalize your blood pressure, it will probably reduce the amount of medication you need.

The main problem though is not that lifestyle changes don't help. The problem is that most people don't sustain them. It is hard to lose weight and keep it off. Salt is ubiquitous in our diet, and it is hard to maintain the stringent steps needed to avoid it. Exercisers exercise, but nonexercisers dabble.

Medication is not a substitute for a healthy diet and exercise. It cannot provide the spectrum of health benefits that the latter does. But there is no doubt that it can bring your blood pressure to target levels that diet and exercise often cannot. **The goal is not to avoid medication at all costs. It is to obtain a normal blood pressure and to do what it takes to get there. The best start is through a healthy lifestyle. But if your blood pressure is still above target, the best path is the right medication, hopefully with the least amount of medication needed to do the job**.

THE ART OF PRESCRIBING

There are now several dozen blood pressure medications to choose from, and numerous choices of combinations and dosages. There is much more to know about the medications than most doctors know, more than any doctor can possibly know.

Although physicians learn a great deal from the medical literature, they also rely on the knowledge acquired from clinical experience. In any specialty, physicians, after treating hundreds if not thousands of patients, discover better ways of prescribing medications, including how to minimize side effects by using the right nuances in doses and in combinations. Over time, they get a sense of what is likely to work, and what is not likely to work for the patient sitting in their room. This type of knowledge is crucial in prescribing wisely.

Different people need different treatment. A drug that works for one patient might do nothing for another. Yet as in many fields, standardized treatment guidelines have taken over and are even imposed, advocating the same basic treatment for all.

The art of medicine goes much further than this. **It is about combining what studies tell us about treating the average patient with what clinical experience teaches us about treating the patient sitting in our office.**

Published treatment guidelines are based on the average response observed in large studies. If 49 percent of people respond to Drug A and only 45 percent to Drug B, guidelines tell us that Drug A is better and that everyone should be treated with Drug A.

That advice is wrong. Many people will respond minimally to Drug A but magnificently to Drug B. For them, Drug B is clearly the better drug, even though, on average, more people will respond to drug A.

Guidelines may tell us that Drug C provides slightly greater protection against heart attack than Drug D. But if Drug D lowers *your* blood pressure much more than Drug C does, it is more likely to protect you from a heart attack and is the drug you need.

The art of medicine is about finding the clues that can tell us which drug is the right fit for you. I hope to communicate many of those clues, as they pertain to the drug treatment of *your* hypertension.

COMBINING PUBLISHED RESEARCH WITH CLINICAL EXPERIENCE

In treating hypertension and many other illnesses, there are two universes of knowledge to call upon: published studies and clinical experience. The medical literature consists of study results, published in peer-reviewed journals. These provide the knowledge from which "evidence-based medicine," the prescription of treatment whose benefit is documented by objective studies, is derived. For example, published studies can tell us that a drug lowers blood pressure. More important, large trials that follow thousands of subjects for a few years can document that lowering blood pressure with that drug actually prevents heart attacks and strokes.

Although "evidence-based medicine" makes sense, unfortunately, the "evidence" is often less reliable than it purports to be. Many studies are sponsored by pharmaceutical corporations, and their design or interpretation may be subject to bias. Many studies are slanted by the financial or intellectual bias of the investigator. An additional problem is that the cost of a large-scale, long-term trial that is now required as definitive evidence of effectiveness in preventing heart attacks and strokes is too great for many excellent, but older or commercially less successful, drugs. As a result, those drugs, no matter how good they are, will never have the "evidence-based" seal of approval.

The other universe of information, clinical experience, provides valuable information not found in the published studies. It doesn't conflict with what studies tell us; it offers guidance regarding questions and issues that have never been examined, and might never be examined, in formal studies. It fills in the gaps in areas where formal studies have not been done, and might never be done.

Many specialists rely on both published studies and clinical observations to refine use of medications. A specialist may notice that some patients require much less or much more than the "usual" dose, or that some do better on different medications than others. Many patients, in a way, have been participants in what is called an "n-of-1" experiment, in essence a single-person experiment, in an effort to find the treatment best suited for him or her. And we apply what we learn over time from patient after patient, to future patients.

Information acquired from formal research is regularly published in medical journals. That which is gleaned from clinical experience rarely is, and usually dies with the practitioner, no matter how skilled and experienced. As a hypertension specialist, I have published many papers concerning my research, as well as some that convey my clinical experience. But many of the clinically valuable and scientifically logical nuances that I have learned will never be published in the journals, because they lack the imprimatur of a formal, published study, with all its regulatory and financial hurdles. I was moved to write this book to communicate what I have learned, which I believe can be helpful in the treatment of many people whose hypertension is not being optimally managed.

The lessons of clinical experience are usually consistent with the results of published studies. But sometimes they aren't. What if clinical experience disagrees with results of published studies? A good study trumps an anecdotal clinical observation. But it would be a grave error to assume that everything researchers report is correct. Although there are many good studies, many other studies are flawed and propagate misleading conclusions. In this regard, when careful and consistent clinical observations stand in glaring opposition to what a study has claimed, a careful look at the study often reveals major flaws in the study.

A PHILOSOPHY FOR PRESCRIBING BLOOD PRESSURE DRUGS

In selecting a drug or drugs for a patient, my philosophy, and the philosophy of many hypertension specialists, is based on the knowledge that in different people, hypertension is driven by different causes. The key to treating your hypertension successfully is to identify the drug(s) and dosage most likely to address its cause or causes.

It would be wrong to prescribe a diuretic ("water pill") to everyone with hypertension. If you have sodium/volume-mediated hypertension (chapter 2), a diuretic would be a good choice. If your hypertension is instead driven by the brain and the sympathetic nervous system, it would not be. As I will explain, there are many clues that can tell us which drug is right or wrong for you, clues that some doctors notice and that many others don't.

A PREVIEW OF THE BOOK

Hypertension and You is organized to make sense of your treatment— which drugs are available, which ones are right for you, and why. To know which medication is right for you, it is first necessary to know what is causing your hypertension and then which drugs address that cause.

The book is organized in the following sequence:

I begin by first discussing the three main mechanisms that cause hypertension (chapter 2). I then identify the drug classes that target those mechanisms and discuss them in the following chapters—how they work and what the side effects are. Moving beyond the standard information, I will provide information that you, and your doctor as well, might not be aware of concerning the drugs you are currently taking or perhaps should be taking. I will identify which are the better drugs, some of which are rarely prescribed, and which are the worst, some of which are best sellers. I will discuss how to avoid or minimize side effects.

In chapter 9, I will focus on the clues that tell us which drugs are likely be right or wrong for you and give tips about individualizing dosage. I will also discuss drug combinations, and how your doctor can select the right combination by deciding which of the three mechanisms to target. I will discuss which combinations make sense and which widely used combinations don't.

The next few chapters help put it all together. I will describe in more detail how you can tell which combinations would be best for you, how to tell if you need higher-than-usual dosage, how resistant hypertension can be brought under control, and how hypertension driven by the mind/body connection can be identified and the different approach needed to bring it under control. I will also discuss the nuances of treatment of hypertension in the elderly.

Finally, I will discuss several areas that are affected by the drug treatment of hypertension: sex, exercise, and safe use of drugs that can raise blood pressure, such as anti-inflammatory drugs and cold remedies. I will also discuss how to reduce or stop medication and how to reduce medication costs.

To sum up, in most cases, hypertension requires drug therapy to achieve a normal blood pressure and maximize protection from cardiovascular events. We are fortunate in that we now have many excellent medications that can, in almost all patients, bring hypertension under control without side effects. Unfortunately, despite doctors' best intentions, millions of patients are on medications, doses, or combinations that are wrong for them. The consequences include inadequate blood pressure control, reduced protection against cardiovascular events, more medications than are needed, avoidable side effects, and unnecessary costs. With the medications available to us today, in almost all cases, if you take your medication, you should expect to have a normal blood pressure, and usually without side effects. You shouldn't settle for less.

1

INCORRECT BLOOD PRESSURE MEASUREMENT AND THE OVERTREATMENT OF HYPERTENSION

It is not an overstatement to say that millions of people are on more blood pressure medication than they need because their blood pressure is measured incorrectly either at the doctor's office or at home. Worse, in most cases, neither the doctor nor the patient is aware that the blood pressure is being overtreated.

In this chapter, I will present the most common errors that doctors make in measuring blood pressure in the office and that patients make in measuring their blood pressure at home. **These errors usually lead to overestimation of blood pressure and to overtreatment.** I will also convey the right way to measure the blood pressure, to avoid readings that are way off the mark.

Blood pressure has been traditionally assessed by measurement in the doctor's office by the doctor or an assistant. Today, however, hypertension specialists and many internists rely more and more on home readings. The studies consistently show that your readings at home are better indicators of risk, and therefore a better guide to the need for treatment, than are office readings.[1] I encourage most of my patients to check their blood pressure at home.

A monitor costs less than $100 and is clearly valuable and cost-effective. For example, you can determine whether or not you have white coat hypertension (i.e., elevated blood pressure in the doctor's office) with normal readings at home. If you do, you might be able to reduce medication and medication costs.

Monitoring your blood pressure at home, you will need fewer visits to the doctor to check your blood pressure, reducing costs for you, for managed care organizations, and for Medicare. Will they reimburse you for the monitor? Probably not, although hopefully that policy is changing!

Another way to assess your home blood pressure is with a twenty-four-hour monitor, with a cuff placed on your arm at the doctor's office and worn for twenty-four hours. Called ambulatory blood pressure monitoring, it is available in the offices of doctors who focus on hypertension. It automatically measures your blood pressure every twenty to thirty minutes over a twenty-four-hour period. It can tell your doctor your average blood pressure and how much it fluctuates. It also assesses your overnight blood pressure, which is at least as powerful an indicator of cardiovascular risk as is daytime pressure. Unfortunately, most health care plans and Medicare won't reimburse the cost, which is usually in the range of $250.

OVERESTIMATION OF YOUR BLOOD PRESSURE AT YOUR DOCTOR'S OFFICE

Table 1.1 lists the most common causes of overestimation of patients' blood pressure in the doctor's office. From what patients tell me, in this era in which doctors of necessity rush to see patient after patient, the most common error doctors make is taking the blood pressure measurement right away. They don't allow you to sit quietly for three to five minutes, as is the standard recommendation, to allow your blood pressure to settle down to its resting level. The result: overestimation of your "resting" blood pressure and overtreatment of millions of patients. It is a huge, yet ignored, problem.

Patients ask me whether the higher reading taken right away reflects a higher risk of developing hypertension or cardiovascular disease. The answer is no, usually not. It is normal for our blood pressure to be higher until we settle down for a few moments.

Table 1.1   Overestimation of your blood pressure at your doctor's office

- "White coat" hypertension
- Failure to sit quietly for a few minutes before the measurement
- Chatting during the measurement
- Wrong size cuff

A second very common cause is chatting during the measurement. Your systolic blood pressure can increase 10 mm or more while talking, enough to affect treatment decisions. I enjoy chatting with patients, but I am rigid in insisting that they sit quietly before I measure their blood pressure. Is it okay if you are quiet and the doctor chats away? Probably.

A third common cause is the use of too small a cuff. If you have a large arm, whether from being overweight or from having a very muscular arm, the usual, standard size cuff might yield misleadingly high readings. A large arm cuff, which every doctor who checks blood pressure should have, solves the problem.

It is recommended that patients be seated in a chair with back support and feet on the ground, rather than on a doctor's exam table with unsupported back and legs dangling in the air. The latter has been reported to produce higher readings.[2] I must confess that I don't follow this recommendation, mainly because when I check the blood pressure in both positions, I find little difference in the readings. So is this recommendation important? I'm not sure.

Other recommendations that are commonly violated are taking a single reading rather than at least three; deflating the cuff too quickly, which will yield a falsely low systolic and falsely high diastolic pressure; and rounding off to the nearest 5 or 10 mm.

The recommendations for how doctors should be measuring blood pressure were recently summarized in a report authored by the late Dr. Thomas Pickering.[2]

White Coat Hypertension

Even if your doctor checks your blood pressure correctly, your readings could still be misleadingly high, a result of the "alerting phenomenon" in the doctor's office. **If your readings are elevated in the doctor's office but are normal elsewhere, you could have what is widely known as "white coat hypertension."**

If your blood pressure is elevated at the doctor's office but is truly normal at home, you are at lower risk of cardiovascular events than if your home readings were also elevated, and you might not need medication. But you must continue to monitor your blood pressure at home to make sure it remains normal, because individuals with white coat hypertension do have an increased risk of developing hypertension in the future.[3] It is okay to ignore the high readings in your doctor's office as long as you monitor your blood pressure at home, at least once a month.

Many patients and doctors wrongly believe that the white coat phenomenon can occur only if a patient feels very nervous when the doctor is checking his blood pressure. That is incorrect. It can also occur in patients who do not feel nervous. That is one more reason to check your blood pressure at home at some point before committing to lifelong medication.

Your doctor's attitude is also an important, widely overlooked factor in white coat hypertension. If your physician fuels your anxiety by telling you "you are a walking time bomb," or "you could have a stroke at any moment," or, even without words, by the alarm he communicates with his facial expression, he can fuel the white coat reaction. By the way, unless your blood pressure is extremely elevated, you are not a walking time bomb.

Another common phenomenon that is not discussed in the medical literature: some patients have elevated readings when they see one doctor and normal readings when they see another. I have seen many patients whose blood pressure is elevated in my office but normal, for example, at their gynecologist. Perhaps it is a result of their focus on blood pressure when they see me. What do I do? I have them check their blood pressure at home, and if the readings are normal, I largely disregard the readings I take.

I also see the opposite: patients whose blood pressure is elevated when they see their general internist and normal when they see me. The alarm that many doctors convey, intentionally or unintentionally, may contribute to this problem. I usually try to be reassuring rather than alarming, in particular because I know that hypertension, if treated wisely, can be controlled in almost everyone and the cardiovascular risk largely eliminated. I believe the reassurance contributes to the lower readings in my office.

OVERESTIMATION OF YOUR BLOOD PRESSURE AT HOME

Some doctors prefer that their patients not check their blood pressure at home, believing the readings might be incorrect or that patients will obsess about their blood pressure. Clearly, some do obsess, and when they do, home readings become uninterpretable. But most people don't, and their home readings are crucial in deciding whether to initiate or increase medication.

However, the readings patients obtain at home are often inaccurate. I would suspect that **millions of people who are checking their blood pressure at home are obtaining misleadingly high readings**. Two of the main reasons are anxiety about their blood pressure and incorrect technique.

Anxiety about the Blood Pressure

Although much attention is given to anxiety-induced elevation of blood pressure in the doctor's office, anxiety while measuring blood pressure at home is also a formidable problem. My experience tells me that many people are nervous when they check their blood pressure at home. In this situation, elevated readings might not be accurately reflecting the usual blood pressure. In the more extreme situation, if a patient tells me he is too frightened to check his blood pressure at home, I don't ask him to check it.

If you are nervous when your blood pressure is checked both at the doctor's office and at home, how can we tell what your blood pressure really is? It can be hard. Wearing a twenty-four-hour blood pressure monitor can often help, although some patients are also nervous wearing that monitor as well.

If you are nervous with office, home, and twenty-four-hour monitoring, it may be impossible to determine what your blood pressure really is, or whether you need medication. In this situation, I monitor for the presence of albumin in the urine or for changes on the echocardiogram as indicators of effects of blood pressure elevation and as a clear-cut indication to treat. I also would err on the side of treating patients who have other cardiovascular risk factors, such as high cholesterol, smoking, diabetes, or overweight.

"Masked" Hypertension

Recent studies focus on the phenomenon called "masked" hypertension, which is the opposite of "white coat" hypertension. Here, the blood pressure is normal in the doctor's office but elevated at home.[4] Since the risk of cardiovascular events correlates more strongly with home readings, "masked" hypertension should be treated, unless the elevated home readings are due to anxiety during the measurement or due to incorrect measurement.

Common Errors That Lead to High Home Readings

Many patients ask me whether the home blood pressure monitors in use are accurate enough. **The problem usually is not the monitors; it is how they are used**. I would suspect that in millions of cases, incorrect measurement technique is contributing to overtreatment. In fact, most of the new patients I see are measuring their home blood pressure incorrectly!

Dos and Don'ts of Measuring Your Blood Pressure at Home

In this section, I will discuss what I believe are the most common errors in home blood pressure measurement (table 1.2). I will also offer guidelines to help you avoid them (table 1.3). Most of the guidelines derive from recently published guidelines for measuring blood pressure at home.[5]

1. Use a monitor with an arm cuff, not a wrist or finger cuff. Studies consistently show that wrist or finger cuffs are not as reliable as arm cuffs.

2. Use an automatic rather than a manual monitor. This recommendation surprises many patients, but, with a manual monitor, the act of pumping the bulb, deflating the cuff at the proper rate, and listening for the sounds, and the effort and hassle of doing it right can affect your blood pressure while you are measuring it. Also, if you are listening for the sounds

Table 1.2   Overestimation of your blood pressure at home

- Checking the blood pressure too frequently
- Checking the blood pressure without first sitting quietly for a few minutes
- Cherry-picking the highest readings
- Inaccurate blood pressure monitor
- Taking single measurements
- Wrong size cuff

Table 1.3   Measuring your blood pressure at home: dos and don'ts

1. Use an arm cuff, not a wrist or finger cuff.
2. Use an automatic rather than a manual monitor.
3. Use a large cuff if you have a large arm.
4. Check your blood pressure in one arm, not both.
5. Sit for a few minutes before checking your blood pressure.
6. When you check your blood pressure, take three readings rather than just one.
7. Don't routinely take more than three or four readings at a sitting.
8. Perform routine blood pressure checks at most twice a week.
9. Check your blood pressure at random times, rather than only when you think it is high.
10. Check the accuracy of your monitor at your physician's office.

with a stethoscope, it is easy to get it wrong. The automatic monitors are not more expensive and are very easy to use. Be sure to use a reliable brand, one certified by the American Association of Medical Instrumentation, the British Hypertension Society, or the European Society for Hypertension. The following website identifies validated brands: www.dableducational .org. On that site, click on "devices" and then "recommended devices." Omron is a reliable brand that I recommend for most patients (I have no financial ties to Omron).

3. Use a large cuff if you have a large arm. If you have a large arm, readings with a regular cuff can be misleadingly high. Ask your pharmacist or doctor if you need a large cuff.

4. Check your blood pressure in one arm, not both. It is a hassle to check both arms. Also the effort of putting the cuff on one arm, measuring the blood pressure, taking it off, and putting it on the other arm can itself keep your blood pressure from settling down.

Another problem is that if you check your blood pressure in both arms, you will usually obtain different readings, not because the blood pressure is different, but because your blood pressure fluctuates from moment to moment. By the time you switch arms, your blood pressure will almost always be somewhat higher or lower.

The arteries in your arms are part of the same circulatory system, and, in more than 99 percent of people, the blood pressure is the same in both arms. In fewer than 1 percent, the readings will differ because of narrowing of an artery in one or both arms from conditions such as severe atherosclerosis or, rarely, inflammatory arteritis. At some point, your doctor should check your blood pressure in both arms to document that the readings are similar. After that, you need not repeatedly check both arms. And if there is a difference between arms, you should be using the arm with the higher reading.

Which arm should you check? It doesn't matter. Choose the arm that's easier to manage. Most right-handed people find it easier to put the cuff on the left arm.

5. Sit for a few minutes after putting on the cuff before checking your blood pressure. This is perhaps the most frequent cause of misleadingly high home readings that I encounter. Many patients report that they put on the cuff and check their blood pressure right away. If you are doing this, you are not measuring your resting pressure. After you put on the cuff, sit for three to five minutes before inflating.

6. When you check your blood pressure, don't take just one reading. Take three readings, about one or two minutes apart. This is another very common error. In many patients, the first measurement is

higher than subsequent measurements. The second and third readings
better reflect your resting blood pressure. The current recommendation
for home measurement is to take three readings and average the second
and third. I strongly recommend doing it that way. If you have waited five
minutes before taking the first reading, it is okay to take the second and
third readings one or two minutes apart (some units come with instructions
to wait for five or ten minutes between readings, which is unnecessary).

   **7. Taking more than three readings can also lead to problems.
Take three readings, record them, and take off the cuff.** When patients take five or ten or more readings, they tend to selectively remember
either the highest or lowest readings. Either tendency provides a misleading picture. If you take reading after reading until you finally get a "good"
reading, or until you work yourself into a frenzy, then the readings become
invalid. On the other hand, if the first three readings vary substantially from
each other, a few extra readings can be helpful in clarifying what your blood
pressure is.

   **8. Check your blood pressure no more than twice a week, unless
you have severe hypertension or are changing medication.** When
a patient of mine tells me that he checks his blood pressure several times
a day, even if he insists that he is not anxious about it, he is. I think some
patients are literally addicted to checking their blood pressure. If you check
your blood pressure five times a day, your concern is probably affecting
your readings, giving you higher, but meaningless, readings. When I encounter patients who do this, I usually ignore the readings. If you cut back,
and check your blood pressure less often, your readings might fall dramatically. The tough part: it can be tough cutting back.

   **9. Check your blood pressure at random, ordinary times, not just
when you "think it is high."** If you check your blood pressure only when
you think it is high—for example, when you are very anxious or angry or upset—you are in essence cherry-picking your highest readings. Many people
do this. Your blood pressure is of course higher at these times. These temporary, and normal, elevations are not representative of your usual blood
pressure. Pick random times to check your blood pressure, some days in the
morning and some days in the afternoon or evening. If you want to know
what your blood pressure is when you are upset, you can check it, but don't
make a habit of doing that.

   10. Check the accuracy of your monitor at your doctor's office.
Don't assume your home monitor is accurate. You need to have it checked
perhaps once every year or two. Your doctor, or the office nurse or technician, can validate it against a manual cuff.

Use Your Monitor to Gather Information—
Do Your Own Experiments

Home blood pressure monitoring gives you a fabulous opportunity to perform your own experiments to determine what elevates your blood pressure and what doesn't. You can assess the effects of a low- versus high-salt diet (give it a few days), cold remedies, anti-inflammatory drugs, coffee, and anything else you want to check.

For example, does caffeine raise your blood pressure? In some people, it does; in others, it doesn't.[6] With self-monitoring, you can determine whether it does or doesn't. It is simple: after checking your blood pressure, drink one or two cups of coffee, and recheck your blood pressure one or two hours later. You can also determine whether the effect is small (less than 5 mm) or larger (more than 10 mm). Of course blood pressure can always fluctuate randomly, so, for greater certainty, repeat the experiment on a few different days.

FREQUENTLY ASKED QUESTIONS

With more and more patients monitoring their blood pressure at home, a number of questions come up again and again. Here are some.

Am I at Risk of a Stroke If My Blood Pressure Suddenly Shoots Up?

Are sudden increases in blood pressure dangerous? Will a sudden increase cause a stroke?

First, let me reassure you that it is normal for our blood pressure to fluctuate. It can be normal one minute and very high the next. A sudden increase is extremely unlikely to cause sudden harm. Except in the rarest cases, nothing at all will happen to you if your blood pressure rises from 120 to 200. **Most people have occasional readings above 200, even if they never had hypertension.** When I run, my blood pressure is likely to be 180 or higher. During weightlifting, someone who has never had hypertension can have readings of 230/120 or higher!

It is your *usual* blood pressure that is much more important than the occasional blip. If your usual blood pressure level is elevated, that is a problem. The occasional blip usually isn't, unless it is very severe, or is associated with physical symptoms, or unless you have a condition for which even normal blood pressure fluctuation is potentially dangerous (e.g., a dissecting aneurysm).

If your blood pressure is very variable, are you at higher risk than if your blood pressure were consistently normal? The answer to this question is still debated. What then should you do if your blood pressure tends to fluctuate? The answer depends on what your usual blood pressure is. The occasional blip is not a problem. But if your blood pressure is elevated on and off and your average blood pressure is increased, yes, you clearly are at higher risk.

Which Is More Important, Systolic or Diastolic Blood Pressure?

For decades, researchers and doctors focused on diastolic pressure as the more important. (In the reading 120/80, 120 is the systolic and 80 the diastolic). However, it is clear that the risk of stroke or heart attack is more closely related to the systolic pressure.[7, 8] Large trials have consistently shown this.

What Level of Blood Pressure Should Be Treated? To What Level Should the Blood Pressure Be Brought Down?

Currently, the goal for blood pressure measured in the doctor's office is a systolic pressure below 140 (below 130 for those with diabetes or kidney disease) and a diastolic pressure below 90, preferably below 80. For readings measured at home, the goals are 5 to 10 mm lower. In general, I aim for an office systolic pressure below 130 in most patients.

In patients over the age of eighty, the goal is less clear. The HYVET study (Hypertension in the Very Elderly Trial) proved that lowering the systolic pressure below 160 is beneficial, but no study has assessed whether lowering it further to below 140 confers extra benefit, or harm.[9] I usually aim for a systolic blood pressure below 140; but I would not add drug after drug to get there, at least until there is clear proof of benefit.

Why Does My Blood Pressure Increase and Stay Up for Days, Seemingly for No Reason? Do I Need More Medication?

Many patients with well-controlled hypertension occasionally experience elevated readings for a few days or even a week or two. When this happens, many think they have become "immune" to the medication, a phenomenon that by the way does not happen. Most doctors respond by increasing dosage or adding another medication, which is how some people gradually end up on more and more medication.

I disagree with this practice; if there is no reason for your blood pressure to be higher, and it is left alone, it will usually fall back to its usual level, by itself, within a week or two. A week or two of mild blood pressure elevation has negligible risk. The main harm occurs if your blood pressure remains elevated for years or decades. Remember also, if your home blood pressure averages, for example, about 120/80, by definition you will have moments or days with lower and higher readings.

What causes the temporary elevation? Severe stress can cause a temporary increase. And sometimes it's a mystery. But I believe the most frequent cause is an increase in sodium intake. Here the blood pressure will usually come back down by itself. In patients who are taking a diuretic, if this happens frequently, I often recommend temporarily increasing the diuretic dose, as I discuss in chapter 3. The dose can then be reduced once the blood pressure is back down and sodium intake is back to its usual level.

If, on the other hand, your blood pressure increases and remains elevated, particularly above 160 or so, you might truly need a change in medication. But even then, imminent danger is very unlikely.

The take-home point: **if your blood pressure is usually well-controlled, your medication should not be permanently increased every time you or your doctor notices an elevated reading.** It is best to follow your blood pressure for several days and give it a chance to fall by itself. And if you need an increase in medication, the need might be temporary. If, however, the elevation is severe, or you don't feel well, or you have an underlying condition for which mild elevation is a problem, then it should be brought to your physician's attention, and an increase in medication might be needed.

People do not become "immune" to blood pressure medication. However, your blood pressure can creep up and stay up, for example, if you gain weight or increase your sodium intake, or simply with aging. In other words, a persisting increase in your blood pressure can occur when new factors have come into play. Here an increase in medication may be needed.

Is Blood Pressure Elevation Caused by Physical Activity a Problem?

Our blood pressure normally increases during physical activity, but this elevation is not harmful. In fact, regular exercise leads to a lower blood pressure, improves longevity, and protects against heart attack and stroke.

Can the increase in blood pressure during exercise ever cause harm? Actually, yes, the temporary elevation in heart rate and blood pressure can increase our cardiovascular risk in the moment. For example, it can increase the chance of rupturing a "vulnerable" plaque in a coronary artery. Despite this, the benefit of exercise, in terms of reducing cardiovascular risk at all other times, greatly outweighs the momentary risk of harm, which is why exercise is so unanimously recommended by doctors.

Is Blood Pressure Reactivity to Stress Harmful to Us?

During stress, our blood pressure increases and then falls back to its baseline. Even if you don't have hypertension, stress can increase your systolic blood pressure to 180 or higher.

People with an exaggerated blood pressure response to stress are called "hot reactors." Studies are divided as to whether or not hot reactors are at increased risk of developing hypertension or of suffering cardiovascular events.

If your blood pressure is perfectly normal but you are a hot reactor, should you be put on medication? To date there is no proof of benefit. However, here I would recommend monitoring your blood pressure for a twenty-four-hour period to see what your average blood pressure is during the day and night. If it is high once in a while, but on average is normal, I would leave it alone. If it is elevated again and again throughout the day, and significantly elevates your average blood pressure, I would consider drug treatment.

Many patients ask me whether a stressful life, or day-to-day stress, leads ultimately to hypertension. Researchers have been trying for decades to prove that it does, but have been unable to do so. I recently published a review of studies on job stress: most studies did not find that job stress caused hypertension.[10]

Then does hypertension have a mind/body connection? I believe that in some cases it does but that the connection is very different from what you probably think it is, as I discuss in chapter 11.

Although stress doesn't cause hypertension, it can increase your risk of heart attack. If there is vulnerable plaque in your coronary artery, transient blood pressure elevation during stress can, in the moment, increase the risk of plaque rupture, causing a heart attack.

2

FINDING THE DRUGS THAT ARE RIGHT FOR YOU

Targeting Three Mechanisms That Underlie Hypertension

The drug treatment of hypertension has become increasingly complicated. There are several dozen antihypertensive drugs to choose from, too many for most doctors to know well. Some doctors habitually prescribe to all their patients only a small handful of drugs that they are most familiar with. Or they might prescribe a new drug with starter samples left by a pharmaceutical rep. But too often, drugs are selected without any specific rationale.

My philosophy in treating hypertension has two cornerstones (table 2.1): (1) **No one treatment fits all**. Each patient has to be treated as an individual. (2) **Each patient should be treated with the drug or drugs whose mechanism of action matches the mechanism underlying his or her hypertension.** Different patients need different drugs, depending on the mechanism(s) causing their hypertension. With this approach, treatment is actually not that complicated.

The basis of my approach is that **in most cases, hypertension is driven by one or more of only three mechanisms** (table 2.2). Focusing on

Table 2.1   Principles of drug selection

1. No one treatment fits all. Different patients need different drugs and doses.
2. The best drugs for *you* are those that match the mechanism(s) underlying *your* hypertension.

Table 2.2   The three mechanisms that underlie hypertension, and the drugs that target them

Mechanism	Drug classes
Sodium/volume	Diuretics, CCBs
Renin-angiotensin system (RAS)	ACEIs, ARBs, DRIs, beta-blockers
Sympathetic nervous system (SNS)	Beta-blockers, alpha-blockers, central alpha-agonists

these three mechanisms can greatly simplify, and make sense of, the task of picking the right drug(s). By selecting and combining drugs that attack one, two, or, if needed, all three of these mechanisms, hypertension can be controlled in almost everyone. It sounds simplistic, but it works. I rely on this approach in my practice, particularly with patients with hard-to-control hypertension. And I have written about it in hypertension journals.

In this chapter, I will briefly describe these three mechanisms and the drug classes that address them. In chapters 3 through 8, I will go through the drug classes, focus on the problems with how they are prescribed, and present better ways to prescribe them. I will identify what I believe are the best and worst drugs. I will tie it all together in chapter 9 by describing the clues that help tell us which mechanisms are probably driving your hypertension and which drug or drug combination would be the best fit for your hypertension. Then, in chapter 10, I will present the strategies I use, as a hypertension consultant, in treating patients with "resistant hypertension," whose hypertension has not been controlled by multidrug therapy.

THE THREE MAIN MECHANISMS THAT UNDERLIE HYPERTENSION

The three mechanisms that underlie hypertension are actually built into us for good reasons: **we need them to keep our blood pressure from falling too *low*.** We'd be dead without them. But when they go somewhat awry, they cause high blood pressure. And when that happens, we need treatment for hypertension, ironically aimed at these same mechanisms.

Sodium/Volume

One cannot read a newspaper without reading about the high sodium content of our diet. The high sodium intake raises blood pressure, minimally in some and substantially in many others. It increases blood pressure both by expanding our blood volume, and by increasing the sodium and calcium content of arterial smooth muscle cells, causing our arteries to constrict.

Our bodies have two defenses that prevent excessive sodium from increasing our blood pressure. One is excretion of sodium through our kidneys. The other is relaxation of our arteries. If we don't excrete the excess sodium, or if our arteries fail to relax in the presence of excess sodium and volume, our blood pressure will rise.

A relative excess of circulating sodium and volume contributes to hypertension in half or more of patients with hypertension. It is a particularly common cause of hypertension in African-Americans, whose kidneys, more often than in whites, are genetically programmed to hold on to sodium. Ironically, this genetic programming originally helped survival in populations living in a tropical climate and consuming a natural low-sodium diet, in whom there was a need to hold on to sodium. But in a temperate climate with a high sodium intake, this survival advantage is instead considered a "genetic defect," because holding on to sodium is responsible for volume-mediated hypertension.

Excess sodium also commonly contributes to hypertension in the older population, due to the kidneys' reduced efficiency in excreting it. Individuals with reduced kidney function due to kidney disease are also prone to "volume-mediated" hypertension.

Volume-mediated hypertension responds best to treatment with a diuretic (chapter 3) or a calcium channel blocker (chapter 4).

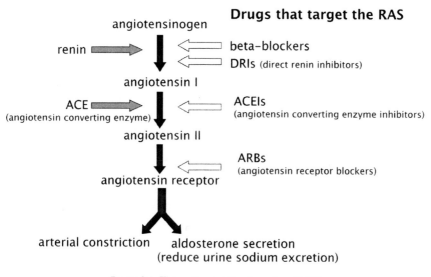

Figure 2.1 The renin-angiotensin system (RAS)

The Renin-Angiotensin System (RAS)

The RAS is a hormonal system that helps keep our blood pressure from falling too low. Normally, it is stimulated when our blood volume or pressure is low, and suppressed when it is high.

The system's sensors are in the kidneys. When our kidneys sense that our blood volume or blood pressure is on the low side, they increase their secretion of the hormone renin, which triggers the system (figure 2.1). Renin enters the bloodstream and catalyzes the formation of angiotensin I, which in turn is converted by angiotensin-converting enzyme (ACE, for short) into **angiotensin II**. **Angiotensin II** binds to and activates angiotensin receptors with many effects but two in particular that raise blood pressure:

- Angiotensin II constricts arterial walls.
- Angiotensin II stimulates secretion of the hormone aldosterone by the adrenal glands, which causes the kidneys to retain rather than excrete sodium.

Stimulation of the RAS keeps our blood pressure from falling below normal. But if it is stimulated when blood pressure and volume are not low, it can lead to high blood pressure.

If the RAS is at least partly responsible for your hypertension, then blocking it can lower your blood pressure. In chapters 5 and 6, I discuss **the four drug classes that antagonize the effect of the RAS on blood pressure: the angiotensin-converting enzyme inhibitors (ACEIs), angiotensin receptor blockers (ARBs), the direct renin inhibitors (DRIs), which are the newest drug class, and the beta-blockers.** As shown in figure 2.1, each antagonizes the RAS at a different point in the system, but they share the same common result: antagonism of the RAS.

The Sympathetic Nervous System (SNS)

The SNS, which sends nerves from our brain to various parts of our body, provides second-to-second control of our blood pressure. A low blood pressure will stimulate it. It is also stimulated when we need an increase in blood flow and/or blood pressure, such as during exercise. But overactivity of the SNS, when not needed, can cause unwanted blood pressure elevation.

A simplified version of the SNS makes it much easier to understand what it does to our blood pressure and how antihypertensive drugs antagonize those effects. It is easiest to look at the SNS as having two limbs, the **adrenal limb** and the **neural limb** (figure 2.2). These two limbs stimulate what are called alpha- and beta-adrenergic receptors (alpha- and beta-receptors for short), which affect the state of contraction of the heart and arteries.

The Adrenal Limb of the SNS   The nerves of the **adrenal limb** of the SNS descend from the brain down the spinal cord, ending in the adrenal glands, which they stimulate to secrete the hormone **adrenaline** into the bloodstream. Adrenaline stimulates both **alpha- and beta-receptors**, but **mostly the beta-receptors,** in our heart and arteries.

Stimulation of **beta-receptors** in the heart causes it to beat faster and more forcefully, increasing the amount of blood pumped into the arterial system (cardiac output) and elevating mainly the systolic blood pressure. When we have a burst of adrenaline, such as from fear or excitement, sometimes we can feel our heart pounding. Stimulation of beta-receptors in the walls of our arteries causes them to relax, allowing increased blood flow.

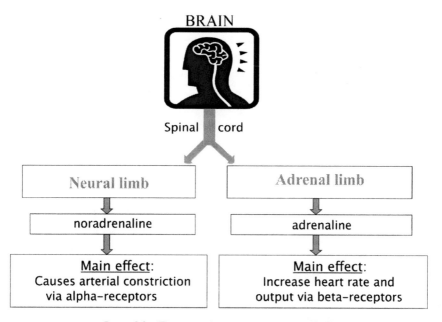

Figure 2.2   The sympathetic nervous system (SNS)

By both increasing heart rate and relaxing arterial walls, adrenaline increases blood flow and cardiac output, which is just what we would want a burst of adrenaline to do during a physical challenge. That is why adrenaline is considered the "fight or flight" hormone.

The Neural Limb of the SNS   The nerves of the **neural limb** of the SNS descend down our spinal cord and terminate in the walls of our arteries and in the heart. The nerve endings secrete the hormone **noradrenaline**, which also stimulates both alpha- and beta-receptors, but **mostly the alpha-receptors** in arterial walls, causing the arteries to constrict, resisting blood flow and raising blood pressure.

SNS Stimulation   The SNS is activated by physical and by emotional stimuli. Usually both limbs, adrenal and neural, are stimulated, although one is usually stimulated more than the other, depending on the stimulus. Fear, for example, stimulates mainly the adrenal limb, with an often dramatic increase in heart rate. Lifting a heavy weight stimulates mainly the neural limb. Some stimuli (e.g., anger) raise blood pressure through both limbs, increasing both heart rate and arterial constriction.

It is through the SNS that emotions affect our blood pressure. Many people don't realize that **it is normal for emotional stimuli to transiently elevate our blood pressure.** Our blood pressure increases when we are frightened or angry or upset, and then returns quickly to normal. That is not hypertension; that is a normal response to emotion.

Most hypertension experts believe that the effects of the SNS on blood pressure are temporary and do not lead to persisting hypertension. That view is shifting, as some experts are beginning to accept that in some patients, the SNS is very much an underlying mechanism of hypertension. Many physicians though don't consider the SNS when they are selecting a drug for your hypertension.

I believe that the SNS is the driving force of hypertension in about 15 percent of cases, and that in most cases of SNS-driven hypertension, it is emotions that are driving the SNS and the hypertension. Unfortunately, the mind/body connection is a greatly underrecognized and, I believe, greatly misunderstood cause of SNS-mediated hypertension. I believe the mind/body connection is very different from that which most doctors and patients believe, and that the understanding of this connection is crucial in selecting the right medication. In chapter 11, I explain how I believe you can tell whether your hypertension is linked to emotion and, if so, how it can be treated.

The drugs most widely used to address SNS-mediated hypertension are the beta-blockers (chapter 6), the alpha-blockers (chapter 7), and the central alpha-agonists, such as clonidine (chapter 8).

Please keep these three mechanisms—sodium/volume, RAS, and SNS—in mind as we go through the various drug classes in the next few chapters. This understanding will make sense of the medications, and make it much easier for you to understand which drugs are best suited to treat your hypertension and which are not. Some physicians keep them in mind when treating hypertension, but many don't. Too often, the result is the wrong medications and the wrong combinations.

THE ANTIHYPERTENSIVE DRUGS

I have listed the antihypertensive drugs in table 2.3, sorted by drug class. Some drugs that are rarely prescribed are omitted.

In each of the chapters in which the drug classes are presented, I have listed low, average, and high dose ranges for each drug to convey what are conservative and what are aggressive doses. In some instances, those dose ranges will differ somewhat from what is listed in other sources, because in many cases, the original FDA-approved doses are too high or too low. Also, different sources offer different recommended doses.

Throughout the book, I will usually mention drugs first by their generic name and then, in parentheses, by the most commonly used brand name, for example, amlodipine (Norvasc). By convention, generic names are headed by a small letter, and brand names by a capital letter. I will usually specify both names because as drugs come off patent, they are referred to by their generic names, many of which are less widely known than the brand names. For example, you might be more familiar with the brand name Norvasc than with the generic name amlodipine.

Table 2.3   The antihypertensive drugs, classified by drug class

Diuretics (chapter 3)

Long-acting thiazide diuretics
- hydrochlorothiazide (HCTZ) (Hydrodiuril)
- chlorothiazide (Diuril)
- chlorthalidone (Hygroton)
- indapamide (Lozol)
- metolazone (Zaroxolyn)

Short-acting loop diuretics
- furosemide (Lasix)
- torsemide (Demadex)
- bumetanide (Bumex)
- ethacrynic acid (Edecrin)

Potassium-sparing diuretics
- spironolactone (Aldactone)
- eplerenone (Inspra)
- amiloride (Midamor)
- triamterene (Dyrenium)

Combination diuretics: HCTZ with
- spironolactone (Aldactazide)
- triamterene (Dyazide, Maxzide)
- amiloride (Moduretic)

Calcium Channel Blockers (CCBs) (chapter 4)

Nondihydropyridines
- diltiazem (Cardizem)
- verapamil (Calan, Isoptin)

Dihydropyridines
- nifedipine (Procardia)
- amlodipine (Norvasc)
- isradipine (Dynacirc)
- felodipine (Plendil)
- nisoldipine (Sular)

Angiotensin-Converting Enzyme Inhibitors (ACEIs) (chapter 5)

captopril (Capoten)	benazepril (Lotensin)
enalapril (Vasotec)	fosinopril (Monopril)
lisinopril (Prinivil, Zestril)	trandolapril (Mavik)
quinapril (Accupril)	perindopril (Aceon)
ramipril (Altace)	

Angiotensin Receptor Blockers (ARBs) (chapter 5)

losartan (Cozaar)   olmesartan (Benicar)

valsartan (Diovan)   telmisartan (Micardis)

irbesartan (Avapro)   eprosartan (Teveten)

candesartan (Atacand)   azilsartan (Edarbi)

Direct Renin Inhibitors (DRIs) (chapter 5)

aliskiren (Tekturna)

Beta-Adrenergic Receptor Blockers (chapter 6)

metoprolol succinate (Toprol)   bisoprolol (Zebeta)

metoprolol tartrate (Lopressor)   acebutolol (Sectral)

atenolol (Tenormin)   pindolol (Visken)

nadolol (Corgard)   labetalol (Normodyne, Trandate)

propranolol (Inderal)   carvedilol (Coreg)

betaxolol (Kerlone)   nebivolol (Bystolic)

Alpha-Adrenergic Receptor Blockers (chapter 7)

prazosin (Minipress)

doxazosin (Cardura)

terazosin (Hytrin)

Vasodilators (chapter 8)

hydralazine (Apresoline)

minoxidil (Loniten)

Central Alpha-Agonists (chapter 8)

clonidine (Catapres)

guanfacine (Tenex)

methyldopa (Aldomet)

Adrenergic Depleters (chapter 8)

reserpine (Serpasil)

③

THE DIURETICS

Tom, forty-six, was taking four drugs, including a diuretic, yet his blood pressure was still uncontrolled. After I increased the dose of his diuretic, his blood pressure fell to normal and he was able to stop two of the four drugs.

Despite their importance, diuretics, in many ways, are the most underused and misused among the blood pressure drugs. I see cases like Tom's all the time. Millions of people, like Tom, are on more blood pressure drugs than they need, and expensive ones, or have uncontrolled hypertension, because either their doctor did not put them on a diuretic or a high enough dose, or he did not put them on the right diuretic or combination of diuretics. And a lot of patients think of the diuretics as just "water pills" and don't realize that they lower blood pressure just as much as the expensive newer drugs do. **Adjusting the diuretic regimen could bring hypertension under control in half of the millions of people with "resistant hypertension."** Making it trickier though is the

Table 3.1 Common errors in diuretic use that might be affecting you

- You are not on a diuretic, and should be on one.
- The dose you are taking is not enough.
- The dose you are taking is higher than you need.
- You are on a diuretic, and shouldn't be.
- You are not on a potassium-sparing diuretic, and should be on one.

opposite problem: many people with hypertension don't need a diuretic and shouldn't be on one!

There are extremely important nuances in prescribing diuretics (table 3.1), and the medical literature does not provide the guidance that doctors need. Simply prescribing a diuretic does not take care of the "diuretic" part of treatment. The task is to figure out which diuretic or diuretic combination and how much, or whether you need a diuretic at all.

That is why I am devoting this first chapter on the antihypertensive drugs to the diuretics, which are listed in table 3.2. If you are among the tens of millions who are on a diuretic, or should be on one, you will find the chapter very informative and valuable.

In this chapter, I will discuss the three types of diuretics, and how your doctor can best prescribe and combine them. I will discuss the side effects and how to avoid most of them. I will also present a wonderful but virtually unmentioned strategy: varying the dose of the diuretic to match variations in your sodium intake. My patients love this strategy both because it works and because it is hard to avoid salt at all times.

Diuretics are most effective if your hypertension is driven by sodium and volume (chapter 2), and in chapter 9 I discuss the clues that can tell you if your hypertension is in that category. In chapter 10, which discusses resistant hypertension, I will explain how to tell if you need a stronger-than-usual diuretic regimen, and the best ways to strengthen it. I encourage you to raise these points with your physician.

A BRIEF HISTORY OF DIURETIC USE IN HYPERTENSION

Over half a century ago, the advent of diuretics revolutionized the treatment of hypertension. They lowered blood pressure without the severe side effects of earlier drugs, and enabled control of what had previously been uncontrollable hypertension.

In those days, doctors prescribed high doses, typically 100 mg of the commonly used diuretic hydrochlorothiazide (HCTZ), because there weren't any other effective and well-tolerated drugs. Side effects, such as depletion of potassium, were common, but there were no alternatives.

Over time it became clear that much lower doses, such as 25 mg, worked in many patients, particularly when one of the newer antihypertensive drugs was added to it. Then, in the 1980s and 1990s, doctors were discouraged from prescribing diuretics altogether, particularly by drug manufacturers

Table 3.2 The diuretics

	Daily doses (mg)		
	Low dose	Medium dose	High dose
Long-acting thiazide diuretics			
hydrochlorothiazide (HCTZ) (Hydrodiuril)	12.5	25	50
chlorothiazide (Diuril)	125	250	500
chlorthalidone (Hygroton)	12.5 every 2 days	12.5–25	25–50
indapamide (Lozol)	1.25	2.5	5
metolazone (Zaroxolyn)	2.5 every 2 days	2.5–10	20
Short-acting loop diuretics			
furosemide (Lasix)	20	40–80	80–160 twice daily
torsemide (Demadex)	5	10	20–40
bumetanide (Bumex)	0.5	1	2–3
ethacrynic acid (Edecrin)	25	50	100
Potassium-sparing diuretics			
spironolactone (Aldactone)	12.5	25	50–200
eplerenone (Inspra)	25	50–100	100–200
amiloride (Midamor)	5	5–10	10–20
triamterene (Dyrenium)	100	100	200–300
Combination diuretics: HCTZ with			
spironolactone (Aldactazide)	½ of 25/25	25/25	50/50
triamterene (Dyazide, Maxzide)	½ of 25/37.5	25/37.5	50/75
amiloride (Moduretic)	½ of 50/5	½ to 1 of 50/5	50/5

who were promoting newer drugs. The new drugs were expected to prevent heart attacks and strokes better than diuretics did, and with fewer adverse effects. Prescribing diuretics became old-fashioned. Prescribing the expensive new drugs became accepted as the right thing to do, even though many patients could not afford them.

I also began to notice that many patients who were referred to me for uncontrollable hypertension were on every drug but a diuretic. And when I added one, their blood pressure was not hard to control. And few doctors were prescribing a diuretic regimen stronger than 25 mg of HCTZ.

The pendulum finally swung back to diuretic use in recent years, as studies confirmed that diuretics lower blood pressure and prevent strokes and heart attacks pretty much as well as the newer drugs. Their low cost also could not be ignored. And adverse effects were less of a problem at the lower dosage usually prescribed.

The diuretics are now prescribed widely but are still prescribed incorrectly in many patients. How to use them better is the subject of this chapter.

WHICH DIURETIC IS RIGHT FOR YOU?
THE THREE TYPES OF DIURETICS

Diuretics lower blood pressure by increasing excretion of sodium and fluid by the kidneys. This reduces the total body fluid volume and also reduces the concentration of sodium and calcium ions in the smooth muscle cells of the arterial walls, causing arteries to relax rather than constrict, lowering blood pressure.

When you start taking a diuretic, you will have a net loss of sodium and volume over the first few days. You might notice your weight drop a pound or two, or more. After that, your intake and excretion of sodium and fluid usually stay in balance. Otherwise, you would eventually become dehydrated.

There are three types of diuretics (table 3.2): the thiazide diuretics, the loop diuretics, and the potassium-sparing diuretics. The most widely prescribed diuretic for hypertension, by far, is the thiazide diuretic hydrochlorothiazide (HCTZ).

Thiazide Diuretics

The thiazide diuretics act mainly in the distal tubules in the kidneys. Their effect is gradual, and you might or might not notice the increase in urine volume. The two most widely discussed thiazide diuretics are hydrochlorothiazide (HCTZ for short) and chlorthalidone. HCTZ, the most widely prescribed thiazide diuretic, is very inexpensive; I even warn patients about "sticker shock"—they'll be shocked at the low price.

When prescribing a diuretic for hypertension, most physicians, myself included, usually prescribe HCTZ. The usual dose is 25 mg but can range from 12.5 to 50 mg, or even higher. Most doctors prescribe 25 mg and, whether it works or not, stay with that dose.

In many patients, 25 mg is enough. But in others, particularly those with resistant hypertension, it isn't. A recent review by Franz Messerli demonstrates why.[1] His meta-analysis showed that most antihypertensive drugs lower systolic blood pressure, as measured by twenty-four-hour blood pressure monitoring, by an average of about 12 mm, and diastolic, by about 8 (i.e., 12/8). HCTZ at the usual 25 mg daily dose lowers it, on average, by only 8/5. The 50 mg dose does lower blood pressure by 12/5, similar to the other drug classes, but is not commonly prescribed.

Chlorthalidone is usually prescribed at a dose of 12.5 or 25 mg a day or every other day. Its effect lasts one to two days, much longer than the twelve-to-eighteen-hour effect of HCTZ.

Many studies tell us that 25 mg of chlorthalidone lowers blood pressure more than 25 mg of HCTZ does, and is roughly as effective as 50 mg of HCTZ. Long-term trials also indicate that chlorthalidone is as effective as, or possibly more effective than, HCTZ in preventing heart attacks and strokes.[2] Then why do well over 90 percent of doctors usually prescribe HCTZ? Partly force of habit. Also, 25 mg of chlorthalidone causes adverse effects, such as potassium depletion, more frequently than 25 mg of HCTZ does, and in many cases is more than the patient needs. I also strongly believe, as do many others, that the combination of HCTZ with a potassium-sparing diuretic (see below) is preferable to chlorthalidone because it is just as effective and has fewer side effects, but outcome studies using this combination have not been done.

HCTZ versus Chlorthalidone: The Current Controversy and the Third Option

The question of HCTZ vs. chlorthalidone is now being hotly debated in hypertension circles. Which of the two should your doctor prescribe? There is no consensus view. Chlorthalidone is more effective, but the adverse effects are greater.

Here is my approach: For the patient with mild hypertension, and particularly in small or older individuals, I believe 12.5 to 25 mg of HCTZ is often all that is needed, and a stronger diuretic may be overkill. For the bigger patient, or the one with more severe or resistant hypertension, who may need more than 25 mg of HCTZ, there are three options (table 3.3).

Do You Need a Stronger-Than-Usual Diuretic Regimen?

One of the most frequent errors made in managing hypertension is the failure to strengthen the diuretic regimen in patients who need it. In chapter 10, which deals with resistant hypertension, I discuss how you and your doctor can tell if you need a stronger-than-usual diuretic regimen, and the best ways to prescribe it.

Table 3.3   What your doctor can do if 25 mg of HCTZ does not control your blood pressure

> - **If it was ineffective because the dose wasn't enough:**
>   - Increase the HCTZ dose to 37.5 or 50 mg.
>   - Switch to chlorthalidone.
>   - Continue the 25 mg dose and add a potassium-sparing diuretic.
> - **If it was ineffective because your hypertension is not driven by sodium/ volume, and a higher dose won't help:**
>   - Stop the HCTZ and switch to a drug other than a diuretic.

To strengthen the diuretic regimen, the three main options, if your kidney function is normal, are to increase the HCTZ to 37.5 or 50 mg, or to prescribe 25 mg of chlorthalidone, or the third option, which is often overlooked in the midst of this controversy, prescribe the combination of 25 mg of HCTZ with a potassium-sparing diuretic (see below). This combination is more powerful than the HCTZ alone and protects against loss of potassium and magnesium. I usually prefer this option rather than 50 mg of HCTZ or 25 mg of chlorthalidone. No long-term trials have compared the outcome of this combination against that of chlorthalidone alone, but the neutral effect on potassium and magnesium suggests that the benefit would not be less.

Of course if your blood pressure did not respond to 25 mg of HCTZ, there is another possible explanation: your blood pressure elevation is being maintained by the RAS or SNS and not by sodium/volume, and increasing the diuretic regimen is not likely to help and could be harmful. Your doctor should instead add or substitute a nondiuretic drug (see chapter 9).

Adverse Effects of Thiazide Diuretics   The thiazide diuretics work well and are very inexpensive, but have a catch: adverse effects. That is why your doctor should use the lowest dose that works, and, in certain people, even avoid them. Table 3.4 lists the most common adverse effects.

Many patients ask me if diuretics damage the kidneys. They don't. By controlling blood pressure they help protect the kidneys. Often with the loss of fluid caused by diuretics, the blood tests that measure kidney function may look worse, with increases in the blood urea nitrogen (BUN) and creatinine. But these increases reflect elimination of extra fluid, and not kidney damage. Despite the higher numbers, diuretics are a mainstay in the battle to prevent hypertension-induced kidney damage.

Potassium and Magnesium Depletion   Thiazide diuretics increase the urinary excretion of potassium and magnesium, which can lead to weakness,

Table 3.4 Common adverse effects of thiazide diuretics

Potassium and magnesium depletion
Dehydration
Muscle cramps
Erectile dysfunction
Diabetes
Elevated uric acid and gout
Elevated triglycerides
Allergic reactions
Low blood sodium concentration

and rarely heart arrhythmias or kidney damage. Your doctor should check your blood potassium level and kidney function within a month of starting a thiazide diuretic. If it is normal, checking it once or twice a year is usually sufficient.

If your potassium level does fall, the best treatment is to reduce the dose of the thiazide diuretic and/or add a "potassium-sparing" diuretic (see below) to block the loss of potassium in the urine. Eating healthy, high-potassium foods (oranges, cantaloupe, bananas, tomatoes, potatoes, etc.), can also help.

Many patients ask me about potassium supplements. I rarely prescribe them. First, at a low dose of HCTZ, most people don't need one. Second, it can take four to six pills a day to restore and maintain the potassium level. Giving a potassium supplement for thiazide-induced potassium loss is analogous to pouring water into a leaking car radiator. It will continue to leak out. A better way is to stop the leak. And that's what the potassium-sparing diuretics do.

Dehydration   Diuretics can cause dehydration, particularly if you are on a high dose or are consuming very little salt and fluid, for example because of the flu or other illness. Elderly individuals who eat little are also at risk of dehydration and a fall in potassium level. The best way to prevent dehydration is to use the lowest dose that works.

Muscle Cramps   Diuretics can cause muscle cramps, which generally occur at night. We don't really know the cause. Sometimes, they are attributed to potassium and magnesium depletion, but they often occur when potassium and magnesium levels are perfectly normal.

If they are brief and infrequent, and if you need the diuretic to control your hypertension, bear with it. Hopefully your doctor can lower the dose somewhat. Magnesium supplements, such as MagOx 400, might be helpful. Quinine pills were widely prescribed to prevent muscle cramps, and seemed to help, although controlled trials showed them to be minimally effective. As a result, quinine pills are now approved by the FDA only for treating malaria and are much more expensive than in the past. A lower-dose pill is available though over the counter.

If the cramps are a big problem, your doctor can try a different diuretic or replace it with a drug other than a diuretic, such as a CCB. Also, restricting sodium intake can enable diuretic dosage reduction or even elimination of the diuretic.

Erectile Dysfunction (ED)   Diuretics at higher doses, which reduce blood volume and blood flow, can contribute to ED. At lower doses, it is not clear that they do. The topic of ED is discussed in more detail in chapter 15.

Diabetes   Thiazide diuretics increase the likelihood of developing diabetes by about 30 to 40 percent, largely because potassium deficits reduce insulin secretion and effect. If you are at increased risk of developing diabetes, a low dose, or the use of a loop diuretic or potassium-sparing diuretic instead of a thiazide diuretic, reduces the risk of provoking diabetes.

If you developed diabetes while taking HCTZ or chlorthalidone, it is hard to say whether the diabetes was caused by the diuretic or would have developed anyway. What would I do? I'd pick one of the options from table 3.5, emphasize a healthy diet and weight loss, and see if the diabetes resolves.

Elevated Uric Acid and Gout   Diuretics reduce urinary uric acid excretion, increasing the blood uric acid level and the likelihood of developing gout. If you develop gout, switching to a drug other than a diuretic can help prevent recurrences. But if control of your hypertension requires a diuretic, then you need the diuretic.

If gout attacks occur once in a blue moon, you can take an anti-inflammatory drug such as ibuprofen (Motrin) or naproxen (Aleve) to quickly end an attack. If they occur more frequently, your doctor can prescribe a uric

Table 3.5   Thiazide diuretics: how to avoid increasing your risk of developing diabetes

1. Use the lowest dose possible.
2. Combine the thiazide with a potassium-sparing diuretic.
3. Instead of a thiazide, your physician can prescribe either a potassium-sparing diuretic and/or a loop diuretic.
4. Healthy diet, exercise, and weight loss.

acid–lowering drug, such as allopurinol (Zyloprim) or probenecid (Benemid), or the newest drug, febuxostat (Uloric). Taking these pills regularly will lower your uric acid level and prevent attacks. If you truly need a diuretic and develop gout, it is one of the rare circumstances where taking a second drug to combat the side effects of the first, as terrible as it sounds, is the right thing to do.

Elevated Triglycerides   Thiazide diuretics increase the level of triglycerides, a fatty component in the blood. If the elevation is mild, it can be ignored. If extreme, for example, above 400 or 500 mg/dl, it can cause pancreatitis and increase the risk of coronary disease. Here it is best to stop the thiazide diuretic and switch to a loop diuretic or potassium-sparing diuretic, or to a drug other than a diuretic.

Allergic Reactions   An allergic rash can develop; it usually resolves within days or weeks of stopping the drug. Taking Benadryl, 25 or 50 mg up to four times a day, can help, although in severe cases, treatment with corticosteroids may be needed. If you experience an allergic reaction, you should stop the thiazide immediately and contact your physician.

If you are allergic to sulfa-containing antibiotics, should you avoid the thiazide diuretics, which also have sulfa-containing bonds? Many patients and doctors think so, but usually a thiazide diuretic can be prescribed because the sulfa bond is different. In fact, there is no cross-allergenicity between a sulfa antibiotic and a thiazide. However, the fact that you are allergic to sulfa or to any drug means you are allergy-prone, and you are more likely to be allergic to a thiazide diuretic, or to any drug, than someone who is not "allergy-prone."

If you have a history of allergy to sulfa drugs, it is reasonable for your doctor to prescribe a thiazide diuretic, unless your allergic reaction was severe, such as throat swelling or anaphylaxis. An allergic reaction to a loop diuretic or potassium-sparing diuretic is possible, but less likely. The diuretic least likely to cause an allergic reaction is an old, rarely prescribed loop diuretic, ethacrynic acid (Edecrin), a drug unknown to many physicians that is a godsend for patients who need a diuretic and have major allergy problems. Unfortunately, it is rarely prescribed, and is now hard to obtain, and is an example of a drug at risk of disappearing from the market because producing it is not profitable.

Low Blood Sodium Concentration (Hyponatremia)   Thiazide diuretics can lower the blood sodium concentration, a condition called hyponatremia.

Hyponatremia develops mainly in people over the age of seventy who drink a lot of water or other fluids. Thiazide diuretics (and potassium-sparing diuretics) can cause disproportionately more loss of sodium than fluid, which, particularly in individuals who consume a large amount of fluid, results in dilution of the blood sodium concentration.

The normal blood sodium level ranges from 136 to 144 milliequivalents per liter. At 128 to 130, little will happen, but at about 125 or lower, nausea, fatigue, sleepiness, and confusion can occur. Below 120, seizures, coma, and death are possible.

What should your doctor do if your sodium level falls? Two things: First, reduce the dose or stop the thiazide diuretic. Second, instruct you to reduce your fluid intake to less than six glasses a day, and possibly less than three glasses for the first day or two. Even if you stop the thiazide diuretic, you should still avoid excessive fluid intake. **"Eight glasses of water a day" is usually a bad idea.**

If you experienced hyponatremia while taking a thiazide diuretic, many doctors mistakenly assume that you should avoid all diuretics, even if you need one. This is wrong. If you need a diuretic, a loop diuretic, which does not interfere with the excretion of free water, is usually safe, but your doctor must monitor your blood sodium level.

Loop Diuretics

The loop diuretics work more quickly and powerfully than the thiazides. After a dose of furosemide (Lasix), the most widely used loop diuretic, most patients urinate frequently for about six hours (hence the name *Lasix—las*ts *six* hours). You might need to be near a bathroom during those six hours!

A helpful tip that very few doctors suggest: You don't have to take the loop diuretic at the same time every day. Take it when it is convenient for you. If you are going out for a few hours in the morning, take it after you return. But don't take it at bedtime; you don't want to commute to the bathroom all night.

When doctors use a loop diuretic to treat hypertension, they usually prescribe furosemide (Lasix). I prefer torsemide (Demadex). Once-a-day furosemide lowers blood pressure less than the thiazides do because its effect is brief. Taking it twice a day solves that problem but is so ridiculously impractical I rarely prescribe it that way. Torsemide (Demadex) has a slightly longer effect and is more reliably absorbed from the gut. And studies show that **once-a-day torsemide lowers blood pressure as much as the thiazides do.**[3]

Another virtually forgotten loop diuretic, ethacrynic acid (Edecrin), as discussed above, is the relatively unknown diuretic least likely to cause allergic reactions.

When Should a Doctor Prescribe a Loop Diuretic for Hypertension? There are a few circumstances where your doctor should prescribe a loop diuretic rather than a thiazide diuretic (table 3.6). It is more effective than a thiazide in patients with reduced kidney function. It is also preferred, as a more powerful diuretic, in treating patients who have congestive heart failure with fluid retention. A loop diuretic is also a better choice in patients who have had hyponatremia (low sodium concentration), whether or not it was related to taking a thiazide diuretic.

Your doctor might also consider a loop diuretic if you are prediabetic because it is less likely than a thiazide to elevate blood sugar. The loop diuretics also are less likely to lower the potassium level, because of their briefer duration of action.

The Potassium-Sparing Diuretics

The potassium-sparing diuretics lower blood pressure and, unlike the thiazide and loop diuretics, protect against potassium loss in the urine. They stimulate the kidneys to hold on to potassium while excreting sodium in its place. They can be used alone, or can be given in combination with a thiazide or loop diuretic, to treat hypertension and reduce the risk of a fall in potassium level.

There are currently four potassium-sparing diuretics on the market, two of which block aldosterone receptors and two of which act directly in the kidney tubule. Each has specific advantages and disadvantages (tables 3.7 and 3.8).

Potassium-Sparing Diuretics That Block Aldosterone Receptors Aldosterone, a hormone secreted by the adrenal glands when our blood pressure or volume is low, stimulates the kidneys to hold on to sodium and instead excrete potassium. When we take a diuretic such as HCTZ, which causes loss of sodium and volume, our kidneys tend to secrete more

Table 3.6 Situations where a loop diuretic is preferable to a thiazide diuretic

1. If you have congestive heart failure
2. If you have reduced kidney function
3. If you have a history of hyponatremia (low sodium concentration)

Table 3.7   The potassium-sparing diuretics

"Aldosterone receptor blockers"
  spironolactone (Aldactone)
  eplerenone (Inspra)
Drugs with direct effects in the kidneys
  amiloride (Moduretic)
  triamterene (Dyrenium)

Table 3.8   Scorecard: the potassium-sparing agents

	triamterene (Dyrenium)	spironolactone (Aldactone)	amiloride (Midamor)	eplerenone (Inspra)
Cost	$	$	$$	$$$
Side effects	infrequent	**frequent**	infrequent	infrequent
Combination pill with HCTZ	**Dyazide, Maxzide**	**Aldactazide**	**Moduretic**	——

aldosterone. This limits the effect of the diuretic and increases the potassium loss. That is exactly why adding a potassium-sparing diuretic to 25 mg of HCTZ makes more sense than increasing the dose of HCTZ to 50 mg.

Spironolactone (Aldactone), which has enjoyed a resurgence in use in recent years, and the newer eplerenone (Inspra), are the two currently available aldosterone receptor blockers. They are used to treat patients with hypertension and/or heart failure. Many doctors are unaware that it can take up to six weeks to obtain the full effect of spironolactone on blood pressure. It is premature to judge its effect in just one or two weeks, and premature to conclude either that it didn't work or that you need a higher dose.

Either drug can be prescribed alone, or together with a thiazide or loop diuretic. The widely prescribed combination pill Aldactazide contains 25 mg of both HCTZ and spironolactone.

Spironolactone is older and less expensive than eplerenone, but has a number of side effects, particularly erectile dysfunction and tenderness of the breasts (yes, in men), caused by binding to sex hormone receptors. These effects will resolve after stopping the drug for a few weeks. Spironolactone can also cause mild diarrhea or nausea. If your gut doesn't feel right, stop the spironolactone.

Eplerenone (Inspra) and the older amiloride (Midamor), which is an excellent, but underused, potassium-sparing diuretic (see below), have fewer side effects than spironolactone. Eplerenone binds minimally to the sex hormone receptors and is much less likely than spironolactone to cause ED or breast tenderness. A dose of 37.5 to as much as 100 mg of eplerenone is equivalent to the 25 mg dose of spironolactone. Eplerenone is more expensive, and therefore most health plans require a trial of spironolactone first.

Potassium-Sparing Diuretics with Direct Effects in the Kidneys
Amiloride (Midamor) is a terrific old drug that few doctors prescribe or even think of. It is a mild diuretic that lowers blood pressure somewhat, does not lower the potassium level, and usually has no side effects.

Few doctors prescribe it because it was marketed poorly, and at the wrong dose! It is available either as a 5 mg pill, or as a combination pill of 5 mg with 50 mg of HCTZ. There is no 10 mg pill, and few doctors prescribe 10 mg or more, even though many patients need the higher dose. Worse, the combination pill (Moduretic) contains too much HCTZ (50 mg) and too little amiloride (5 mg). We need a 25/5, 25/10, or 50/10 combination pill, but since the drug is old, off patent, and not widely prescribed, that will never happen.

When I prescribe HCTZ and amiloride, instead of prescribing the 50/5 combination pill, I prescribe separate pills, 25 mg of HCTZ with one or two 5 mg tablets of amiloride. If needed, the dose of either or both can be increased. Few doctors do this. If you need more of a diuretic, or need to add a potassium-sparing diuretic, ask your doctor about amiloride, particularly if you have had side effects with spironolactone.

The fourth potassium-sparing diuretic, triamterene (Dyrenium), is combined with HCTZ in two very widely prescribed pills: **Maxzide** and **Dyazide**. I rarely prescribe them because they also contain the wrong dose, too little triamterene, to do the job (37.5 mg with 25 mg of HCTZ, or 75 mg with 50 mg of HCTZ). If I want to prescribe triamterene, I prescribe it as a separate 100 mg pill.

With any of the four potassium-sparing diuretics, there is a risk of excessive elevation of blood potassium level, which can increase the risk of dangerous heart arrhythmia. This is fortunately uncommon, but certain patients are at higher risk of this complication:

- Patients with reduced kidney function
- Patients who are taking a drug that can also increase potassium levels— an ARB, ACEI, DRI, or NSAID (nonsteroidal anti-inflammatory drug, such as ibuprofen [Motrin] or naproxen [Aleve])

If you have reduced kidney function or are taking other drugs that increase potassium levels, a potassium-sparing diuretic should be used with caution or even avoided. And checking your potassium level is a must.

Would a Potassium-Sparing Diuretic Be a Good Option for You?

Table 3.9 lists four situations in which a potassium-sparing diuretic is a very good idea. If you had a low potassium level on a thiazide diuretic, adding a potassium-sparing diuretic will usually restore it to normal while further lowering your blood pressure. If 25 mg of HCTZ did not control your hypertension, adding a potassium-sparing diuretic, instead of increasing the dose of the HCTZ or taking 25 mg of chlorthalidone, can lower your blood pressure without increasing potassium loss.

Your doctor can also prescribe a potassium-sparing diuretic by itself, instead of a thiazide—for example, if you are allergic to a thiazide or are diabetes-prone. Finally, a potassium-sparing diuretic is the diuretic of choice in patients whose hypertension is caused by an excess of the hormone aldosterone (see chapter 12).

FLEXIBLE DIURETIC DOSING: A LOGICAL YET RARELY USED STRATEGY

The "Morning-After" Pill

Day after day, I encounter patients whose blood pressure increased after they consumed more salt than usual, typically through salty restaurant food when eating out or when on vacation or on a business trip.

Almost everyone's salt intake varies, and published studies have not addressed what to do about the blood pressure variation that it often causes.

Table 3.9   When your doctor should consider prescribing a potassium-sparing diuretic

---

- **Your physician might add a potassium-sparing diuretic if:**
  - your potassium level fell on HCTZ.
  - 25 mg of HCTZ did not control your blood pressure.
- **Your physician might prescribe a potassium-sparing diuretic by itself if:**
  - you have a history of allergic reaction to a thiazide.
  - you are diabetes-prone.
  - your potassium level fell with a thiazide.
  - your hypertension is caused by an excess of the hormone aldosterone (chapter 12).

Here's the dilemma: prescribing a high daily dose of a diuretic might be too much when your salt intake is low; prescribing a lower daily dose might be too little when your salt intake is high.

It seemed pretty logical that my patients could benefit from a higher dose when splurging on salt, and a lower dose at other times. I call it a "morning-after" pill. I began advising patients to do this. For example, I might instruct a patient to take 25 mg when eating out and 12.5 mg when eating at home, or 37.5 mg (a pill and a half) instead of their usual 25 mg. I found that the blood pressure was controlled better and that patients loved this approach—they know they cannot follow a low-salt diet at all times.

I suggest that you discuss this strategy with your doctor, to eliminate faster the excess sodium and retained fluid.

Although what I call "flexible dosing" is an obvious strategy, I have not seen it discussed in any study or textbook, and know few doctors who do this. But it is so logical that even in the absence of formal studies, I recommend it and suggest that you discuss it with your doctor.

Finally, the issue of flexible dosing has an important flip side. I recommend reducing the dose, or even stopping the diuretic, if you are consuming much less salt than usual—for example, if you have the flu and are not eating. Common sense dictates that if you are eating next to nothing and taking in little or no salt, you have less need for the diuretic.

HOW TO STOP A DIURETIC

Another issue that is seldom discussed is how to stop a diuretic. When we take a diuretic over a period of time, the loss of sodium and fluid stimulates our kidneys to try to hold on to salt and fluid. If we then stop the diuretic, our kidneys, still geared up to try to hold on to sodium and fluid, and now unopposed by the diuretic, will cause retention of a few pounds of fluid for a week or two or longer. You will feel bloated and may have edema (fluid) in your legs. This is one reason why I try to prescribe the lowest diuretic dose possible, to minimize the tendency to retain sodium and fluid.

Patients and their doctors often interpret this fluid retention as proof that they need to go back on the diuretic. Sometimes they do. But often they don't; with time the extra fluid will come off by itself.

How can you prevent the bloating and fluid retention when stopping a diuretic? Stop it gradually. I advise patients to taper, from a pill a day to half a pill, and then to a half every other day, each reduction at least a week apart. This allows the body to adjust gradually to the withdrawal of the diuretic.

WHICH IS BETTER: SALT RESTRICTION
OR A DIURETIC?

If your hypertension is driven by salt and volume, restricting salt intake can lower your blood pressure, but you have to be diligent, aiming for less than 2,000 mg of sodium a day, or, even better, 1,000 mg. By comparison, the average American consumes over 3,500 mg. **If salt restriction lowers your blood pressure to normal, you can avoid medication. If it doesn't, then you need medication. But even then, it can reduce the amount of medication you need.**

Most people are unaware of how much sodium is in their food. They think their sodium intake is low if they don't add salt at the table, but table salt is actually the least of our sodium intake. Most comes from restaurant food, processed food, and foods with high sodium content, with a large contribution also coming from baked goods such as bread, rolls, and bagels.

The most reliable method for assessing your sodium intake is measurement of the sodium contained in a twenty-four-hour urine collection. Few doctors ask patients to do this. If you want to know how much sodium you are taking in, ask your doctor for this test. In my research, I am working on a method to estimate twenty-four-hour sodium excretion from just a sample of urine, and I hope this will greatly simplify the procedure.

THE BOTTOM LINE

If your doctor is prescribing a diuretic for your hypertension, which should he prescribe, and how much?

1. Usually a thiazide, such as HCTZ or chlorthalidone, at a low or medium dose (see table 3.2), depending on your size, on your sodium intake, and on how high your blood pressure is. Chlorthalidone, a less widely used alternative, is equal to or superior to HCTZ.
2. If you are prone to diabetes and need a diuretic, a loop diuretic (my favorite is torsemide [Demadex]) or potassium-sparing diuretic, such as spironolactone (Aldactone), might be preferred.
3. When a regimen stronger than the usual 25 mg dose of HCTZ is needed, I believe adding a potassium-sparing diuretic (spironolactone [Aldactone], amiloride [Midamor], or eplerenone [Inspra]) is preferable to a higher dose of HCTZ by itself. The other alternative is switching to 25 mg of chlorthalidone, but there is an increased risk of developing a low potassium level.

THE CALCIUM CHANNEL
BLOCKERS (CCBs)

How CCB use might be affecting you:

- You suffer from fatigue and are taking a class of CCBs that causes fatigue.
- You suffer from constipation and don't realize that CCBs can aggravate constipation.
- You are retaining fluid in your legs (edema).
- You awaken frequently at night to urinate.
- You are taking a CCB and your blood pressure is not controlled.
- You are on a CCB when you should instead be on a diuretic.

The calcium channel blockers (CCBs) (table 4.1) dilate arteries and are widely prescribed for treating hypertension. Like the diuretics, they tend to work better in patients with sodium/volume-mediated hypertension, and are particularly recommended for black patients, whose hypertension is likely to be sodium/volume-mediated.[1, 2]

The CCBs don't affect the potassium, sodium, and glucose levels. Since they lack these adverse metabolic effects that often accompany diuretic use, many believed they would be better at preventing atherosclerosis. This led many physicians to prescribe CCBs instead of diuretics. However, long-term studies showed that the diuretics controlled blood pressure and prevented strokes and heart attacks pretty much as well, and at a fraction

Table 4.1 The calcium channel blockers

	Daily doses (mg)		
	Low dose	Medium dose	High dose
Dihydropyridines			
nifedipine (Procardia)	30	30–60	90
amlodipine (Norvasc)	2.5	5–10	10
isradipine (Dynacirc)	2.5 twice daily	5–10 twice daily	10 twice daily
felodipine (Plendil)	2.5	5	10
nisoldipine (Sular)	20	20–40	60
Nondihydropyridines			
diltiazem (Cardizem)	120	240–360	420
verapamil (Calan, Isoptin)	120	240–360	480

Combination pills :

amlodipine + an ACEI or ARB:
amlodipine + benazepril (Lotrel)
amlodipine + valsartan (Exforge)
amlodipine + olmesartan (Azor)
amlodipine + telmisartan (Twynsta)
amlodipine + aliskiren (Tekamlo)

amlodipine + an ACEI or ARB + a diuretic:

amlodipine + valsartan   + HCTZ (ExforgeHCT)
amlodipine + olmesartan   + HCTZ (Tribenzor)

amlodipine + aliskiren   + HCTZ (Amturnide)

of the cost. And CCBs do have side effects that many users are living with. In this chapter, I will describe the two subclasses of CCB and to whom I would prescribe them.

THE TWO TYPES OF CCB: DIHYDROPYRIDINE AND NONDIHYDROPYRIDINE

The two main subclasses of CCBs are:

Dihydropyridine CCBs (e.g., amlodipine [Norvasc], nifedipine [Procardia]).

Nondihydropyridine CCBs (e.g., verapamil [Calan], diltiazem [Cardizem]).

These two subclasses differ considerably from each other. The **dihydropyridine CCBs** relax and dilate the arteries with virtually no effect on the heart. The two most widely prescribed dihydropyridine CCBs are amlodipine (Norvasc) and nifedipine (Procardia). The short-acting form of nifedipine, which lasts only four to six hours, is no longer used.

The **nondihydropyridine CCBs** relax the arteries, though not as powerfully, and also slow the heart rate. The two nondihydropyridine CCBs—verapamil (Calan, Isoptin) and diltiazem (Cardizem)—are a particularly nice fit if you have hypertension and a rapid heart rate. Studies indicate that they lower blood pressure as much as the dihydropyridine CCBs do, but in my experience, the dihydropyridines often lower blood pressure more.

DRUG COMBINATIONS

The CCBs are often used in combination with other antihypertensive drugs. There are now many combination pills on the market that combine amlodipine with either an ACEI or an ARB (table 4.1). CCBs can also be given along with a beta-blocker, with the CCB dilating arteries and the beta-blocker reducing the heart rate and output. A word of caution: nondihydropyridine CCBs (diltiazem and verapamil) should usually not be combined with a beta-blocker because both drugs lower the heart rate. CCBs are also given in combination with a diuretic, although combining them with a diuretic might lower blood pressure less than combining them with an ACEI or ARB.[3]

SIDE EFFECTS

If you are taking a CCB, there are several side effects you could be experiencing without realizing that the drug is the cause. Several side effects are common to all the CCBs:

Edema, (fluid retention) in the legs, occurs in about 10 to 15 percent of people taking a CCB. You might notice the indentation above your socks

Table 4.2   CCB side effects

- **All CCBs**
  - Edema (fluid retention in the legs)
  - Constipation
  - Increased urinating at night
- **Dihydropyridine CCBs**
  - Headaches
  - Palpitations
  - Overgrowth of gums
- **Nondihydropyridine CCBs**
  - Fatigue

and the tightness in your shoes at the end of the day. It is not dangerous but can be bothersome. If you tended to have edema before starting a CCB, the edema might worsen. That is why I usually try to avoid CCBs in patients who have edema.

The edema in turn is responsible for another side effect: **increased urination at night**, caused by reentry of fluid from the legs back into the bloodstream, when off one's feet overnight. Another frequent side effect, seen more commonly with the nondihydropyridine CCBs, is **constipation,** which can be severe, particularly in older patients. Diuretics can also cause constipation but usually not as much. **If you are on a CCB and suffer from constipation, ask your doctor to try changing your medication.** There are enough alternatives that you need not aggravate this problem.

The **dihydropyridine CCBs** can also cause **headaches** and/or **palpitations**. The headaches, which are not dangerous, usually cease after a day or two. If they continue to occur, it is best to change medication.

Some patients taking a dihydropyridine CCB experience a somewhat increased heart rate, a result of slightly increased sympathetic nervous system tone that occurs in response to dilated arteries. If it is bothersome, switching to verapamil or diltiazem will solve the problem.

Finally, an odd side effect is overgrowth of the gums. This can sometimes lead to the need for surgical intervention unless the drug is stopped.

The **nondihydropyridine CCBs** verapamil and diltiazem, which slow the heart rate, don't cause palpitations or headaches but do cause **fatigue** in many patients. I prescribe them infrequently because of this. **If you are taking a nondihydropyridine CCB and your energy is less than it was, you should ask your doctor about switching to a different drug.**

DIHYDROPYRIDINE OR NONDIHYDROPYRIDINE: WHICH IS BETTER FOR YOU?

Because of the fatigue issue, I almost always prescribe a dihydropyridine, such as amlodipine (Norvasc) or nifedipine (Procardia). I prescribe a nondihydropyridine (verapamil or diltiazem) in patients who have a rapid heart rate, or who developed a headache or allergic reaction while taking a dihydropyridine CCB.

5

THE ACEIs, ARBs, AND DRIs

Targeting the Renin-Angiotensin System

I am discussing the ACEIs, ARBs, and DRIs together because each lowers blood pressure by antagonizing the effects of the RAS (chapter 2). The beta-blockers also antagonize the RAS but are discussed separately in chapter 6 (tables 5.1 and 5.2).

Your blood pressure will generally respond equally well to an ACEI, ARB, or DRI. If one lowers your blood pressure, any of the others usually also will. And if one doesn't lower your blood pressure, the others probably won't either. In other words, if your doctor tried an ACEI or ARB and it did nothing, you are better off switching to a different drug class whose target is not the RAS.

THE ACEIs, ARBs, DRIs, AND BETA-BLOCKERS

The ACEIs, ARBs, DRIs, and beta-blockers antagonize the RAS, but at different points (figure 5.1).

Table 5.1 The four drug classes that antagonize the RAS

- Angiotensin-converting enzyme inhibitors (ACEIs)
- Angiotensin receptor blockers (ARBs)
- Direct renin inhibitors (DRIs)
- Beta-blockers

Table 5.2   Drugs that target the RAS

	Daily doses (mg)		
	Low dose	Medium dose	High dose
Angiotensin-converting enzyme inhibitors (ACEIs)			
captopril (Capoten)	12.5 twice daily	25–50 twice daily	100–150 twice daily
enalapril (Vasotec)	5	10–20	40
lisinopril (Prinivil, Zestril)	5	10–40	80
quinapril (Accupril)	5	10–40	80
ramipril (Altace)	2.5	5–10	20
benazepril (Lotensin)	5	10–40	80
fosinopril (Monopril)	10	10–40	80
trandolapril (Mavik)	1–2	2–4	8
perindopril (Aceon)	4	4–8	16
Angiotensin receptor blockers (ARBs)			
losartan (Cozaar)	25	50–100	100 twice daily
valsartan (Diovan)	40–80	80–160	320
irbesartan (Avapro)	75	150–300	300
candesartan (Atacand)	8	16–32	32
olmesartan (Benicar)	5	20–40	40
telmisartan (Micardis)	20	20–80	80
eprosartan (Teveten)	400	600	800, or 400 twice daily
azilsartan (Edarbi)	40	80	80
Direct renin inhibitors			
aliskiren (Tekturna)	75	150–300	300

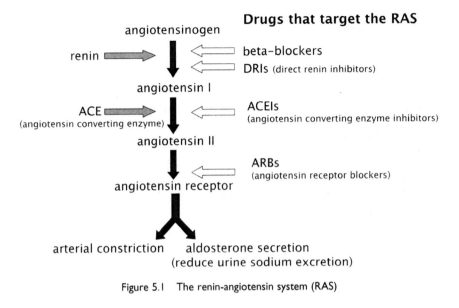

Figure 5.1   The renin-angiotensin system (RAS)

The beta-blockers inhibit secretion of renin; the DRIs block renin from binding to its receptor, preventing formation of angiotensin I. The ACEIs bind to ACE, preventing conversion of angiotensin I to angiotensin II. And the ARBs occupy and block the angiotensin receptors, preventing angiotensin II from binding to and activating those receptors. **Although the four drug classes operate at different sites, their effect is pretty much the same: inhibition of the RAS.**

The DRI is the newest and most expensive of these drug classes. The only DRI on the market, aliskiren (Tekturna), is worth using if you've had an allergic reaction to an ACEI or ARB, but otherwise there is no data yet to indicate that it is worth the extra cost. In this chapter, I will focus on the ACEIs and ARBs, which are the two most widely prescribed anti-RAS drugs.

ACEIs and ARBs

Your doctor doesn't need to be familiar with all of the available ACEIs and ARBs, because, with only a couple of exceptions, one lowers blood pressure pretty much the same as another. But there are some differences to be aware of.

Choosing among the ACEIs   There are a few differences among ACEIs. Captopril must be taken twice a day, the others usually once a day.

All of the ACEIs except fosinopril (Monopril) are eliminated from the body by the kidneys. Their dose should be reduced in patients with reduced kidney function. Fosinopril (Monopril), eliminated by both liver and kidney, doesn't require dosage reduction.

Choosing among the ARBs   The ARBs also differ little from one to another, with the possible exception of the oldest ARB, losartan (Cozaar), which may be less effective and may have a shorter duration of effect than the others.[1, 2] In some patients, losartan may need to be taken twice a day. Losartan is the only ARB that lowers the blood uric acid level, although the effect is small and probably not relevant.

Studies show that the newest ARB, azilsartan (Edarbi), which appeared on the market in 2011, lowers blood pressure more than the other ARBs.[3] It is not yet clear why. In patients with uncontrolled hypertension, I sometimes switch from a different ARB to azilsartan instead of adding another drug.

Cost   The cost of ACEIs and ARBs depends mainly on whether generic versions of the drug are available. Generic versions are available for the older ACEIs but not for the newer ones. They are pretty much as effective as the brand name ACEIs, and prescribing them reduces medication costs.

What about the ARBs? Here it is a little trickier: studies show that the first ARB to go generic, losartan (Cozaar), is less effective than other ARBs,[1, 2] and I am reluctant to switch patients from other ARBs to losartan. Fortunately, generic versions of more ACEIs and ARBs are becoming available.

Many health care plans also dictate that your doctor switch from one branded ACEI or ARB to a different one. Most of the drugs are equally effective, so usually it is okay to switch.

Which Is Better for You: An ACEI or an ARB?   Should your doctor prescribe an ACEI or an ARB? They are about equally effective, in terms of blood pressure control and prevention of heart attack and stroke. About 10 percent of people who take an ACEI develop an annoying cough and end up switching to an ARB. If you develop the uncommon allergic reaction of angioedema (swelling in the facial and throat area) while taking an ACEI or, more uncommonly, an ARB, your doctor should switch you to a DRI.

If ACEIs and ARBs lower blood pressure by the same amount, and ACEIs cause a cough, why not start everyone on an ARB? At the moment there is only one reason: cost. More ACEIs than ARBs are available as generic versions. Since there is a 90 percent chance that you won't develop a cough with an ACEI, the cost saving of a generic ACEI over a brand name ARB makes sense. As generic ARBs become available, the advantage will switch back to the ARBs.

Can an ARB Be Added to an ACEI?   Yes, but since both block the same mechanism, the RAS, combining them will not lower your blood pressure much more than either by itself. Studies show that the combination of an ACEI and ARB lowers systolic blood pressure only 2 mm more than either by itself, and also, that the combination does not protect against heart attack or stroke any better than either by itself.[4] In other words, you gain very little from combining them. If you are on an ACEI, for example, your blood pressure will fall much more if your doctor adds a diuretic or CCB than if he adds an ARB. As a rule of thumb, combining a diuretic with an ACEI or ARB will almost double the amount by which your blood pressure is lowered, from 12 mm to 20–25. If your doctor has you on both an ACEI and an ARB, you can usually stop one or the other and save the cost.

One circumstance in which we do combine an ACEI and ARB is if you have kidney disease and increased protein in the urine. The combination reduces loss of protein more than either drug by itself and might help slow the worsening of the kidney disease.

Side Effects of ACEIs and ARBs   ACEIs and ARBs are generally very well tolerated. But there is an important, yet seldom emphasized, problem that can occur with the first dose: if you take the first dose when your blood volume is low, either from a very low salt diet or a diuretic, your blood pressure can fall too much, causing weakness or faintness. The antidote is usually to lie down and consume something salty. You should also contact your physician.

To prevent this problem, when I prescribe an ACEI or ARB to a patient who is on a very low salt diet or on a diuretic, **I often recommend skipping the diuretic for a day or two, and/or taking the first dose with a salty meal.** Patients love it—a salty meal on doctor's orders!

Several patients who came to me with hard-to-control hypertension told me they could not take an ACEI or ARB because when they had tried one, it lowered their blood pressure too much. That actually tells me that the ACEI or ARB worked and might be exactly the drug they need. The problem is simply that it worked too well because their blood volume was a little low when they started it. I would restart the drugs, at lower dosage and perhaps with a salty meal.

Uncommonly, an ACEI/diuretic or ARB/diuretic combination causes a large increase in the blood creatinine and blood urea nitrogen (BUN) levels, indicating reduced kidney function. There are two possible causes, one benign and one very serious. The benign cause: the combination was too strong and somewhat reduced blood perfusion to the kidneys. Your doctor can remedy this problem by reducing the dosage of one or both drugs, and then repeating the blood tests to make sure they return toward baseline. This generally does not lead to permanent damage.

The more serious situation is when the sudden reduction in kidney function is a result of severe narrowing in the arteries that supply both kidneys (chapter 12). Here the kidney function might not return to baseline until the ACEI or ARB is stopped. In these cases, tests to determine whether the arteries to the kidneys are blocked should be done to determine whether repair of the artery is needed (chapter 12).

If your kidney function worsens on an ACEI or ARB, it might be unclear whether it is the benign or serious cause. Your doctor might need to screen for blockage in the arteries to the kidneys, even if the kidney function returns to normal after stopping the drug. Your doctor should suspect this problem particularly if you have severe hypertension, have been a lifelong smoker, or have a very high cholesterol, all of which lead to atherosclerotic narrowing of arteries.

Side Effects of ACEIs   COUGH   The most common side effect, which occurs in about 10 percent of cases, is a dry, annoying cough, a sense of tickling in the throat. It is harmless, in most cases, but annoying.

Actually it *can* be harmful if your doctor doesn't realize the ACEI is the cause and orders all kinds of tests and x-rays, looking for a cause, rather than first stopping the ACEI to see if that solves the problem. Also, many patients with a cough fail to mention it to their doctor, and suffer for months. If you don't mention it, your doctor won't do anything about it.

Surprisingly, the cough can first develop even after years of taking an ACEI. Here both you and your doctor might not think the ACEI is the cause. Be aware that it might be.

If you develop a cough on an ACEI, tell your doctor. He should stop the ACEI and can replace it with an ARB. The cough will resolve within a few days. If it doesn't, then your doctor should consider other causes.

ANGIOEDEMA   ACEIs more so than ARBs uncommonly cause an allergic reaction called angioedema. It consists of swelling in the face, mouth, and/or throat, or elsewhere. Uncommonly, it can obstruct breathing, which is why it is important to stop the drug immediately if you develop any facial swelling.

Fortunately, only 1 or 2 percent of patients who take an ACEI experience angioedema, and only a small proportion of those who do run into serious problems. If you develop the swelling, stop the drug immediately and call your physician. If your breathing is becoming difficult, get to an emergency room. And be aware, angioedema can develop for the first time even after years of taking an ACEI or ARB.

If you develop angioedema with an ACEI or ARB, your doctor should switch you to the DRI aliskiren (Tekturna) or to a drug from a different drug class, anything other than an ACEI or ARB.

Side Effects of ARBs   The ARBs are extremely well tolerated, with a side effect rate very close to that of a placebo. That's why the ARBs are such a great drug class. One potential adverse effect, as with ACEIs, is excessive lowering of blood pressure with the first dose, particularly in patients who are taking a diuretic, as discussed above. Also, rarely, an ARB can cause angioedema.

A recent paper that concerned a number of my patients reported that ARB use was associated with an increase in the risk of developing cancer.[5] However, as has been the case with cancer scares involving other antihypertensive drugs, a subsequent larger study found that ARBs are not associated with cancer.[6]

Direct Renin Inhibitors (DRIs)

Aliskiren (Tekturna)   Aliskiren is the only available DRI. Its effect lasts two days, offering a slight advantage over ACEIs and ARBs in that if you miss a dose, your blood pressure will remain under control a little longer.

Since aliskiren targets the RAS, if your blood pressure responded to an ACEI or ARB, it is likely to respond to aliskiren as well. If it didn't, it probably won't. What about combining aliskiren with an ACEI or ARB? Since they affect the same system, the combination is not likely to lower your blood pressure much more than either by itself. Valturna, which combines the ARB valsartan (Diovan) with the DRI aliskiren (Tekturna), does lower systolic blood pressure more than either alone, but only by 4 mm.[7] Worse, a recent study, which has not yet been published, found that this drug combination does not provide more protection against heart attack or stroke than either drug by itself; if anything the risk might be slightly higher! As a result, Valturna was removed from the market, and in the future, there is unlikely to be any support for combining an ACEI or ARB with a DRI.

The main use for aliskiren is in patients who need an RAS blocker but are allergic to an ACEI or ARB. Otherwise, it is usually not worth the higher cost. When the price comes down, it might deserve equal footing with ACEIs and ARBs, although long-term studies are needed to confirm that it prevents heart attacks and strokes as well as the ACEIs and ARBs. It probably does.

Beta-Blockers

Beta-blockers, which I discuss at length in the next chapter, attack two of the three mechanisms of hypertension: the RAS and the sympathetic nervous system (SNS). When the goal is to block the RAS, an ACEI or ARB is usually preferable to a beta-blocker both because they provide better protection against heart attack and stroke[8] and because they don't have the many side effects that beta-blockers do (chapter 6). However, there are some patients in whom a beta-blocker is the right drug, as I also explain in the next chapter.

I encounter many patients who are on a beta-blocker and don't need to be on one. If you are on one for the purpose of antagonizing the RAS and are experiencing side effects such as fatigue, ask your doctor if he could switch you to an ACEI or an ARB instead.

BETA-BLOCKERS

When They Are Necessary and When They Aren't

THINGS YOU MIGHT NOT KNOW ABOUT TAKING A BETA-BLOCKER

- For most people with hypertension, a beta-blocker is the wrong drug!
- Beta-blockers given for hypertension are causing fatigue in millions of people, most of whom don't really need to be on a beta-blocker!
- You might not realize you lack pep on a beta-blocker until you stop it (don't stop it without consulting your physician).
- Many people who are on a beta-blocker are suffering avoidable side effects because they are on too high a dose, or are on the wrong beta-blocker.
- If you feel tired on a beta-blocker, your doctor can usually do something about it. You don't have to live with it.

Millions of people are taking a beta-blocker for hypertension (table 6.1). Most don't know that beta-blockers provide less protection than ARBs or ACEIs do against heart attack and stroke,[1] and cause more side effects than do most other antihypertensive drugs. The most common side effect: fatigue.

They also don't know that **most people suffering fatigue from a beta-blocker taken for hypertension don't really need to be on the beta-blocker! Frankly, for most people being treated for hypertension, a**

Table 6.1 The beta-blockers

	Daily doses (mg)		
	Low dose	**Medium dose**	**High dose**
metoprolol succinate (Toprol)	25	50–100	200–400
metoprolol tartrate (Lopressor)	25 twice daily	50–100 twice daily	200 twice daily
atenolol (Tenormin)	12.5	25–50	50–100 twice daily
nadolol (Corgard)	20	40–80	240
propranolol (Inderal LA)	60	80–160	160
betaxolol (Kerlone)	¼ of 10-mg tab	¼, ½, or 1 10-mg tab	20
bisoprolol (Zebeta)	½ of 5-mg tab	½ or 1 5-mg tab	10
acebutolol (Sectral)	200	200–400	800
pindolol (Visken)	½ of 5, twice daily	½ or 1 5-mg tab twice daily	10 twice daily
labetalol (Normodyne, Trandate)	100 twice daily	100–300 twice to three times daily	400 three times daily
carvedilol (Coreg)	3.125 twice daily	6.25–25 twice daily	25 twice daily
carvedilol CR (Coreg CR)	20	20–80	80
nebivolol (Bystolic)	2.5	5–10	20–40

beta-blocker is the wrong drug! And if you need a beta-blocker, there are ways to avoid or lessen side effects.

Beta-blockers are responsible for millions of people feeling tired, lacking pep, every day! And many of them don't even realize that it is the drug that is making them tired. They think it is just part of aging. Or they got used to it and don't realize how much pep they are lacking. Or they just feel lazy.

Many are suffering from other side effects as well, such as cold hands and feet, erectile dysfunction, thinning hair, and others. These are not life-threatening but make life a bit worse for the many years that people take them.

Then why do doctors still prescribe beta-blockers so widely, and how can we use them better? **Should you be on a beta-blocker for your hypertension?** Are some tolerated better than others? That's what this chapter is about.

Most doctors believe that one beta-blocker is the same as another. They aren't. There are *hugely* important differences in terms of both effectiveness and side effects. By the end of this chapter, you will know a lot more about those differences.

In this chapter, I will explain how beta-blockers work and will review their good and bad features. I will clarify who should and shouldn't be on one. I will discuss their side effects, and what you and your doctor can do about them. I will discuss the differences among the beta-blockers and identify which ones I believe are better than others.

Beta-blockers are also prescribed to treat conditions other than hypertension, such as coronary heart disease, heart arrhythmias, and heart failure. This discussion is not directed at those conditions.

HOW DO BETA-BLOCKERS LOWER BLOOD PRESSURE?

"Beta-blockers," or, more correctly, "beta-adrenergic receptor blockers," bind to beta-receptors in the kidneys and in the heart (and in other sites). They prevent "beta-receptor agonists" (activators), particularly adrenaline, from binding to and stimulating those receptors, preventing the effects that can elevate blood pressure (table 6.2).

Beta-blockers antagonize two of the three hypertension mechanisms that we have discussed (chapter 2): the **renin-angiotensin system (RAS)** and the **sympathetic nervous system (SNS).** Specialists argue about which of these two effects is most responsible for lowering blood pressure. My belief is that, in most people, it is the effect on the RAS that is responsible for blood pressure lowering, and that to antagonize the RAS, an ACEI or ARB is a better choice than a beta-blocker. I also believe that hypertension is driven by the SNS in about 15 percent of cases, and here, a beta-blocker,

Table 6.2 Three mechanisms by which beta-blockers can lower blood pressure

1. They suppress the renin-angiotensin system (RAS).
2. They block effects of the sympathetic nervous system (SNS).
3. They reduce anxiety.

often combined with an alpha-blocker (see chapter 7), is incredibly effective in lowering blood pressure and is the right drug. Finally, I will also discuss a third, often ignored effect through which beta-blockers lower blood pressure: their antianxiety effect.

The Renin-Angiotensin System (RAS)

When beta-receptors in the kidneys are activated, they stimulate secretion of the hormone renin, which activates the RAS and raises blood pressure (chapter 2). **Beta-blockers suppress the secretion of renin, reducing activation of the RAS and lowering blood pressure.** The ACEIs, ARBs, and DRIs (chapter 5) also antagonize the RAS, and if your hypertension is driven by the RAS, one of these drugs is usually preferable to a beta-blocker because they provide better protection against cardiovascular events and have fewer side effects.[1]

The Sympathetic Nervous System (SNS)

As discussed in chapter 2, the SNS increases our blood pressure through two effects: a) it increases heart rate and output through stimulation of beta-receptors in the heart and b) it constricts arteries through stimulation of alpha-receptors in the artery walls. Beta-blockers prevent adrenaline from increasing our heart rate and cardiac output, but lack the desired effect of reducing arterial constriction. This is why I usually prescribe an alpha-blocker along with the beta-blocker, to address the vasoconstriction. This is an incredibly effective, yet very underused, drug combination, as I discuss in chapter 7.

Antianxiety

There is a third, often ignored mechanism: the antianxiety effect of beta-blockers. When we are anxious and secreting adrenaline, we feel our heart pounding and feel tremulous and sweaty. These physical sensations often feed our anxiety, causing us to secrete yet more adrenaline and feel more anxious, creating a vicious cycle. The adrenaline increases our heart rate and systolic blood pressure.

Beta-blockers prevent the heart pounding and tremulousness, making our anxiety less likely to spiral. We are feeling less anxious, our SNS is stimulated less, and we secrete less adrenaline. This is why beta-blockers are widely and successfully used in lessening stage fright. They also slow down our heart rate.

I often prescribe a beta-blocker in hypertensive patients who seem "wired" and have a rapid heart rate, to kill two birds with one stone. It lowers the increased heart rate and often reduces the anxiety, which tamps down the SNS, lowering the blood pressure. That is why I am inclined to start treatment of hypertension with a beta-blocker by itself in tense, "wired" people. In many cases, patients feel better with it and it is the right drug for them.

Interestingly, in my experience, some patients who are generally fatigued from their tenseness actually feel more energetic on a beta-blocker! I have occasionally prescribed a beta-blocker for patients with chronic fatigue, and some feel better.

How can one tell whether a beta-blocker is the right or wrong drug? Will it cause fatigue or lessen it? The answer is simple: the patient will tell me whether it is the right or wrong drug for him, by reporting how he feels on it. If he feels fatigued, it might be the wrong drug. If he feels better, it is exactly the right drug.

IF YOU NEED A BETA-BLOCKER, WHICH ONE IS BEST FOR YOU?

Many doctors are unaware of the important differences among beta-blockers with regard to both effectiveness and side effects. If you are on the wrong beta-blocker, it might not be doing the job or might be causing avoidable side effects. I will devote the coming pages to explaining this and to picking and choosing among the beta-blockers.

KEY DIFFERENCES AMONG BETA-BLOCKERS

There are many differences among the beta-blockers, and a few of those differences, which are listed in table 6.3, have extremely important effects with regard to effectiveness and side effects.

Whether or Not a Beta-Blocker Is Metabolized by the Liver

Beta-blockers are absorbed by the intestine and pass through the liver before entering the bloodstream. Some are inactivated in the liver, and some are not (table 6.3).

Table 6.3   Key features that differentiate one beta-blocker from another

---

I. Whether or not the beta-blocker is metabolized by the liver

Beta-blockers that are metabolized	*Beta-blockers that are not metabolized*
metoprolol (Toprol, Lopressor)	atenolol (Tenormin)
propranolol (Inderal)	betaxolol (Kerlone)
labetalol (Trandate, Normodyne)	bisoprolol (Zebeta)
carvedilol (Coreg)	acebutolol (Sectral)
nebivolol (Bystolic)	pindolol (Visken)

2. Beta-blockers that dilate rather than constrict arteries (vasodilating beta-blockers)
  a. Beta-blockers that block both alpha- and beta-receptors
       labetalol (Trandate, Normodyne)
       carvedilol (Coreg)
  b. Beta-blockers with "ISA"
       pindolol (Visken)
  c. Beta-blockers that increase nitric oxide secretion
       nebivolol (Bystolic)

3. Beta-blockers that slow the heart rate less than others (beta-blockers with "ISA")
  pindolol (Visken)
  acebutolol (Sectral)

Beta-Blockers That Are Inactivated by the Liver   Beta-blockers **that are inactivated (metabolized) in the liver are inactivated at different rates in different people.** Determined genetically, some people metabolize them rapidly, and some, slowly. If your liver inactivates them rapidly, very little of the drug will reach your bloodstream and the drug will do little or nothing, even at a high dose. If instead your liver inactivates them very slowly, even a low dose will result in a high blood level, and you will be more likely to experience adverse effects, particularly fatigue.

The blood level that beta-blockers attain can vary ten- to twenty-fold from one person to another, depending on whether one is a fast or slow metabolizer. Unfortunately, there is no widely available test by which to tell.

Also, **beta-blockers that are metabolized by the liver get into the brain more than others do.** A slow metabolizer will have a high blood level and with it a high brain level. This can contribute to fatigue and mental dullness, and, particularly in the case of propranolol, depression and nightmares.

Beta-Blockers That Are Not Inactivated by the Liver The blood level of these beta-blockers is more predictable and differs less from one person to another. That is why I prefer to prescribe them, particularly the relatively ancient betaxolol (Kerlone) and bisoprolol (Zebeta).

Vasodilating versus Vasoconstricting Beta-Blockers

Unlike most other antihypertensive drugs, most beta-blockers constrict rather than relax small arteries. This reduces blood flow through them, contributing to unwanted effects such as cold hands and feet, an increased risk of developing diabetes, erectile dysfunction, hair thinning, and others. Whew! Most hypertensionists agree that a beta-blocker that dilates arteries would seem preferable. I will discuss the vasodilating beta-blockers later in this chapter.

Beta-Blockers That Slow the Heart Rate Less Than Others

When beta-blockers occupy beta-receptors and block out adrenaline, the heart rate can fall to the 50s, or even lower. Two beta-blockers, pindolol (Visken) and acebutolol (Sectral), have "intrinsic sympathomimetic activity (ISA)," and slightly stimulate the beta-receptors while occupying them. The main advantage of this is that the heart rate doesn't fall as much; the heart rate will slow down to 60, not 50 or 40. Of the two I prefer pindolol because the smallest acebutolol capsule contains 200 mg, which is too much. Pindolol is a pill that can be broken in half to provide a smaller starting dose.

Many doctors are unaware of pindolol, which is most useful in patients who had developed a very slow heart rate on other beta-blockers. It is also my impression that patients feel less fatigued on pindolol, although I am not aware of any studies that have examined this.

A BRIEF TOUR OF THE BETA-BLOCKERS

I believe the differences between beta-blockers, which are not widely appreciated, are important enough to review the most widely prescribed beta-blockers one by one. I will also discuss some beta-blockers that I believe should be, but aren't, widely prescribed.

In this section, I will briefly describe their advantages and disadvantages. If you are on a beta-blocker, you should be aware of these important differences.

Atenolol (Tenormin) **Advantages:** Atenolol, the second best-selling beta-blocker, is not metabolized by the liver, so the blood level is more predictable. Generic atenolol is very inexpensive.

Disadvantages: In some people, atenolol does not last twenty-four hours unless it is given twice a day. It is unclear whether the once-a-day dosage provides as much protection against cardiovascular events as do other beta-blockers.

Best use: Atenolol is inexpensive, but its effect doesn't always last twenty-four hours, which is disadvantageous for long-term cardiovascular protection. Some patients need to take it twice a day.

Betaxolol (Kerlone)   Few physicians have heard of betaxolol, and even fewer prescribe it. It is one of my favorite beta-blockers. **It might be the most reliable beta-blocker in terms of blood level and effect**.

If it is so good, why do so few physicians prescribe it? Bad marketing. It could and should have been a best seller. Instead, it creeps along with dismal sales and is sometimes hard to obtain. I'll be happy if this book improves its sales. (No, I have no financial ties to betaxolol.)

Advantages: Number one is the predictable blood level and effect. Also, betaxolol is among the longest-acting beta-blockers, lasting up to two days. Its effect persists even if a dose is forgotten. It provides a very consistent blood level throughout the day and night rather than having a very high peak level followed by a very low level twenty-four hours after the dose.

Disadvantages: A minor disadvantage is that the smallest pill, 10 mg, is more than most people need. I start most patients on half a pill (5 mg) or even a quarter of a pill (2.5 mg) once a day, leaving them with the nuisance of having to break the pills.

Best use: I prescribe betaxolol more than any other beta-blocker when I am treating patients for whom I believe a beta-blocker is the right drug for their hypertension. It is an excellent beta-blocker.

Bisoprolol (Zebeta) **Advantages:** Like betaxolol, bisoprolol is not metabolized by the liver and provides a very reliable blood level. Also, like betaxolol, it was not marketed successfully.

Disadvantages: Like betaxolol, the lowest dose pill, 5 mg, is more than many people need. I start many patients on just half of a pill.

Best use: Bisoprolol, like betaxolol, is one of my favorites when I feel a beta-blocker is the right drug.

Metoprolol (Toprol, Lopressor)   Metoprolol, the best-selling beta-blocker, is one of my least favorite. Its prominent sales are a testament to great marketing. Almost every cardiologist I know automatically selects Toprol. Most medical residents also select Toprol, foreshadowing its continued wide use.

Advantages: There is nothing unique about metoprolol that justifies its number-one position on the market. It does reduce mortality in patients with heart failure, but there is no reason to believe that this is unique among beta-blockers.

Disadvantages: Metoprolol and other beta-blockers that are metabolized by the liver provide an unpredictable blood level, often too low or too high. Also, drug entry into the brain can cause fatigue and mental dullness.

Best use: I don't believe metoprolol has any unique advantages to justify its being the number-one seller. The shorter-acting form is useful in the hospital when quicker onset and offset of action are desired.

Propranolol (Inderal) **Advantages**: Propranolol, the oldest beta-blocker, is helpful for stage fright. It works within an hour and wears off within hours. It is also available as a longer-acting once-a-day pill.

Disadvantages: Because of high drug levels in the brain, it can cause nightmares and depression. Propranolol is metabolized by the liver, and its blood level is unpredictable.

Best use: For stage fright, the relatively quick onset and offset of action make propranolol a good choice. Otherwise, there is probably no reason to prescribe it.

Vasodilating Beta-Blockers

Most of the beta-blockers cause constriction of small arteries. However, there are now three types of beta-blockers that dilate rather than constrict small arteries (table 6.3): beta-blockers with alpha-blocking effects (alpha-blockers are discussed in chapter 7), beta-blockers with intrinsic sympathomimetic activity (ISA), and beta-blockers that increase nitric oxide secretion.

Beta-Blockers with Alpha-Blocking Effects Labetalol (Normodyne, Trandate) and the newer carvedilol (Coreg) block both beta- and alpha-receptors. Blocking the alpha-receptors dilates small arteries (chapter 7), improving blood flow through them.

Carvedilol (Coreg) **Advantages:** Carvedilol, by blocking alpha-receptors, also dilates arteries. In diabetics, carvedilol, unlike metoprolol, does not worsen glucose levels.[2]

Disadvantages: Like labetalol (Trandate, Normodyne) and metoprolol (Toprol), carvedilol is inactivated by the liver, and the blood level is unpredictable. The generic form of carvedilol is taken twice a day; the newer carvedilol CR is taken once daily, but is more expensive.

Best use: Carvedilol may be preferable over metoprolol in hypertensive patients who have diabetes or congestive heart failure. However, because of the unpredictable blood levels, if I want both alpha- and beta-blockade, I prefer prescribing the alpha- and beta-blockers as two separate drugs to provide a more predictable blood level (chapter 7).

Labetalol **Advantages:** Labetalol is available as a pill and also as a liquid for intravenous injection for treatment of hypertensive crises. It is safe in pregnancy and is widely used in pregnant women and in nursing mothers.

Disadvantages: Labetalol is inactivated in the liver, and therefore provides unpredictable blood levels. In addition to the usual beta-blocker side effects, it also causes a peculiar tingling sensation in the scalp in about 10 percent of patients.

Best use: Intravenous labetalol for hypertensive emergencies, and oral labetalol for hypertension during pregnancy and in nursing mothers. Otherwise, because of the unpredictable blood levels, if I want the patient to be both alpha- and beta-blocked, I prefer prescribing two separate drugs, a beta-blocker and an alpha-blocker, which provides a more predictable blood level (chapter 7).

Beta-Blockers That Increase Nitric Oxide Secretion

Nebivolol (Bystolic) The newest beta-blocker, nebivolol, blocks beta-receptors and also increases secretion of the vasodilator, nitric oxide, by the lining of arterial walls.

Advantages: Nebivolol dilates rather than constricts small arteries. It may be less likely than other beta-blockers to cause typical beta-blocker side effects such as increased blood sugar levels, fatigue, and erectile dysfunction, although direct comparison studies need to be done to better document this. Also, because of the increase in nitric oxide secretion, nebivolol lowers blood pressure in black patients more than other beta-blockers do. Two patients have reported to me that it reversed hair thinning caused by other beta-blockers, but confirmation in a formal study is needed.

Nebivolol is unique among beta-blockers in another respect: it is metabolized but not inactivated by the liver, so it is more likely to work even in patients who rapidly metabolize it.

Disadvantages: Cost, depending on your drug plan.

Best use: I would consider trying nebivolol in patients who are on a beta-blocker and are experiencing side effects such as fatigue, sexual dysfunction, or hair thinning. It may also be preferable to other beta-blockers in blacks. In the long run, a vasodilating beta-blocker like nebivolol might be preferable in general to the usual vasoconstricting beta-blockers, but long-term studies are needed to prove this.

Beta-Blockers with Intrinsic Sympathomimetic Activity (ISA)

Pindolol (Visken) and Acebutolol (Sectral)   Few doctors are aware of these beta-blockers, and fewer prescribe them. But they have an important niche. When they occupy the beta-receptor, they stimulate it a little, while preventing adrenaline from binding and stimulating it much more. It is analogous to screwing a low-watt lightbulb into a socket, shedding a little light, but preventing anyone from screwing in a high-watt bulb that would produce much brighter light. The mild stimulation causes arteries to dilate rather than constrict, and also lessens the slowing of the heart rate. Typically, the heart rate will be around 60, and not 50 or 40. In my experience, they seem to cause less fatigue than other beta-blockers.

Advantages: They dilate arteries, and cause less lowering of heart rate, and possibly less fatigue, than other beta-blockers.

Disadvantages: Because pindolol and acebutolol have never been big sellers, their manufacturers have not performed the large, expensive long-term studies needed to prove whether or not they prevent heart attacks and strokes as well as other beta-blockers do. Also, pindolol must be taken twice a day.

Best use: I prescribe pindolol in patients who require a beta-blocker, but whose heart rate had fallen below 45 or so on another beta-blocker, particularly if they are experiencing fatigue. (In some cases, the exaggerated fall in heart rate may indicate the need for a pacemaker). I often start with half of the low-dose 5 mg pill twice daily. I prefer pindolol over acebutolol because the acebutolol capsule has too much drug (200 mg) and cannot be broken into half.

IS A BETA-BLOCKER THE RIGHT DRUG FOR YOU?

Because of their side effects, if you don't need to be on a beta-blocker, you shouldn't be on one. Let's go back to the three mechanisms of hypertension that we discussed in chapter 2: **sodium/volume, the renin-angiotensin system (RAS), and the sympathetic nervous system (SNS)**. In about 75 percent or more of cases, hypertension is driven by sodium/volume, the RAS, or both. If it is driven by sodium/volume alone, a beta-blocker usually will not lower your blood pressure, so you shouldn't be on one. If it is driven by the RAS, a beta-blocker is likely to work, but an ACEI or ARB will also work, and are usually a better choice because they protect better against heart attacks and strokes, and have fewer side effects. If your hypertension is attributable to both sodium/volume and the RAS, again, a beta-blocker is not necessary.

Where I use a beta-blocker is in the 15 to 20 percent or so of patients whose hypertension is driven by the SNS, particularly in hypertension driven by the mind/body link (as described in chapter 11 and in my book, *Healing Hypertension* [Wiley 1999]).[3] I prescribe the beta-blocker either alone or together with an alpha-blocker (chapters 7 and 9). I believe this is the niche for which a beta-blocker is best suited.

Why then do doctors continue to prescribe beta-blockers so frequently? Some largely overlook their disadvantages, others are simply accustomed to prescribing them, and continue to do so.

WHY A BETA-BLOCKER MIGHT NOT WORK

Even if your hypertension is driven by the SNS, a beta-blocker still might not work. There are a few possible reasons (table 6.4). If the dose is too low, or if a beta-blocker that is metabolized in the liver is prescribed to someone who is a rapid metabolizer, the blood level of the drug will be inadequate. Or it might not work unless it is given together with an alpha-blocker (chapter 7).

There is an easy way to tell if the dose you are taking failed to provide an adequate blood level: your heart rate. If the beta-blocker didn't slow your heart rate to below 65 to 70 or so, you probably are not "beta-blocked."

Table 6.4   Why a beta-blocker might not lower your blood pressure

- Your hypertension is driven by sodium/volume and won't respond to a beta-blocker.
- The dose you are taking is too low.
- You are a "rapid metabolizer," and the beta-blocker you are taking is metabolized in the liver.
- It won't work unless given along with an alpha-blocker.

SIDE EFFECTS

I was enjoying the company of friends before dinner at our home. Mike, who is sixty, told me his doctor had put him on Toprol for his high blood pressure. I asked if he was experiencing any side effects, and he told me none; he felt fine.

Later, he asked me what kind of side effects might occur. I mentioned fatigue. He slammed his hand loudly on the table. "So that's it!" He had been feeling weak and "draggy." His wife described him as sluggish and grumpy (more than usual). Mike stopped the Toprol and felt much better.

Tens of millions of Americans are on beta-blockers. Many are suffering from side effects that are not trivial (table 6.5)—some realize it and some, like Mike, don't. Worse, **most people taking a beta-blocker for hypertension don't even need to be on one.** Fortunately, if you do need to be on one, you can feel better, either by taking a lower dose or by switching to a different beta-blocker.

I hope this section will lead to a medication change in many, many readers.

Fatigue

I mention fatigue first because it is a frequent problem and may be affecting millions of people. Worse, many will be taking the drug for the rest of their lives. I encounter many patients who think their fatigue is just from laziness or getting older or being a little depressed, never thinking that it might be the beta-blocker they are taking. To put it bluntly, I believe there is **an epidemic of avoidable fatigue**.

Table 6.5   Common side effects of beta-blockers

1. Fatigue
2. Mental/emotional
   a. Mental dullness
   b. Depression
3. Asthma
4. Weight gain
5. Increased likelihood of developing diabetes
6. Erectile dysfunction
7. Hair loss
8. Cold extremities
9. Beta-blocker withdrawal syndrome

Most patients don't develop fatigue while taking a beta-blocker, but some do, and every doctor knows this. I would guesstimate it affects perhaps 10 to 20 percent, many of whom, like Mike, don't even realize they've lost a lot of their get-up-and-go and don't even mention it to their doctor. They might never realize it unless at some point the beta-blocker they are taking is stopped.

Many don't realize they are tired. They *can* do everything they want to; they just don't feel like it. They don't exercise, not because they can't, but because they "just don't feel like it." And being less active, many gain weight. **Beta-blockers are not the friend of people trying to lose weight**.

And many who are tired and gaining weight assume it is because they are depressed, or are just getting older. They don't realize that reducing the dose or changing the drug is all that is needed to restore their vitality.

That said, I also see the opposite. Some patients feel much better on a beta-blocker, particularly those who are wired and have a rapid heart rate. For them a beta-blocker is the right drug. They feel better when a beta-blocker slows down their racing heart and reduces their cardiac output to normal. Again, it is a great drug in the right patient and literally a drag in the wrong patient.

One caution though: **don't stop a beta-blocker without consulting your physician, and certainly don't stop it suddenly.** If you stop a beta-blocker suddenly, a "beta-blocker withdrawal" syndrome can occur, with agitation, a rapid heart rate, risk of heart arrhythmia, and elevated blood pressure. A beta-blocker should usually be tapered over a week or two before being stopped. This should be done under the supervision of a physician.

If you are lacking your normal energy, the beta-blocker you are taking might be the cause. Do bring it to the attention of your physician and insist that he or she not ignore your concern. It is not acceptable for your doctor to ask you to tolerate sluggishness for years.

Mental Dullness

At her first visit with me, Mary did not seem like a very bright woman. I was surprised when she told me she was a corporate executive! She was taking metoprolol (Toprol), and I asked her to taper and stop it. At her next visit, she was like a different person, vital and sharp. It felt like I was meeting her for the first time. It wasn't just my perception. She also realized the profound change.

This often ignored side effect is not fatigue. It is a subtle, or sometimes not-so-subtle, loss of mental sharpness. Some patients who are having this side effect have trouble describing how they feel, but when I comment that patients tell me they feel dull or stupid, the reaction is, yes, that's it. It seems to happen in patients who are taking a beta-blocker that is metabolized by the liver, because those beta-blockers circulate into the brain more than other beta-blockers do, particularly in "slow metabolizers" who have a high blood level. I seem to see it most often with metoprolol probably because metoprolol is the most widely prescribed beta-blocker.

A couple of patients, after I stopped metoprolol, described the effect as feeling like being "let out of jail." The daughter of an eighty-one-year-old patient, after I had switched her mom's medication from metoprolol to the beta-blocker betaxolol (Kerlone), thanked me for "giving me back my mother."

If you are taking a beta-blocker, and you or others have noticed that you seem "duller," I strongly recommend asking your doctor about switching either to a beta-blocker that is not metabolized by the liver or to a drug other than a beta-blocker.

Do Beta-Blockers Cause Depression?

Beta-blockers have been popularly linked to depression, and depression did seem to occur with the first beta-blocker, propranolol (Inderal), which is associated with very high drug levels in the brain. However, for most beta-blockers, formal studies have not confirmed a link with depression.[4]

In my experience, depression is uncommon, but the gamut of beta-blocker side effects—including fatigue, reduced desire to do things, mental dullness, and weight gain—can mimic depression, can readily be confused with depression, and can aggravate it.

Other Side Effects

Other beta-blocker side effects are not trivial and are also affecting millions:

Asthma: It is well-known that beta-blockers can worsen asthma in individuals with a history of asthma. It is not clear how often this happens. As a result, beta-blockers are "relatively" contra-indicated in people with a history of asthma. This means that they can be used with caution in patients who have a history of mild asthma, or a history of asthma in the distant past. In patients with severe or frequent asthma, it is best to avoid the beta-blockers.

Weight gain: Studies confirm a tendency to gain weight while taking a beta-blocker,[5] at least partly because of the subtle reduction in energy and activity. The average weight gain is small, but in my experience, some individuals gain a ton of weight. That is why I try to avoid beta-blockers in overweight patients if their blood pressure can be controlled with other drugs. If a beta-blocker is required, I try to use the lowest dose possible.

Increased likelihood of developing diabetes: Beta-blockers increase somewhat the risk of developing diabetes. Several factors might be responsible: weight gain, reduced exercise, and reduced blood flow through small arteries, which reduces transfer of glucose from blood to muscles.

Erectile dysfunction: By reducing cardiac output and increasing resistance to small artery blood flow, beta-blockers cause ED more frequently than most other blood pressure medications. This might occur less often with the vasodilating beta-blocker nebivolol (Bystolic), but comparative studies are needed.

Cold hands and feet: The constriction in peripheral arteries reduces blood flow to the hands and feet. The extremely common result: cold hands and feet, particularly in cold weather.

Hair thinning: Some women, my guess would be 10 percent or more, notice thinning of their hair. Many don't realize the connection. Again, it is likely a result of arterial constriction with reduced blood flow to the hair follicles. (The opposite occurs with minoxidil, an arterial dilator, which is now available as a hair growth cream.)

How to Avoid or Reduce Side Effects

If you are on a beta-blocker and are suffering from any of the above side effects, here are three strategies that your doctor can use, perhaps with your prodding, to reduce or eliminate them (table 6.6).

My most important recommendation: if you don't really need a beta-blocker, you shouldn't be on one. If your hypertension can be controlled with other drugs, your doctor can switch your medication and

Table 6.6   Three strategies to avoid or reduce beta-blocker side effects

1. If possible, replace the beta-blocker with a drug from a different drug class.
2. If your doctor feels you need the beta-blocker, he should consider reducing the dose.
3. Change to a beta-blocker that is not metabolized by the liver (table 6.3) to avoid excessive blood levels.

taper and stop the beta-blocker. If you do require a beta-blocker, simply lowering the dose can help.

If you are on a beta-blocker that is inactivated by the liver, and happen to be a "slow metabolizer," the blood level might be much higher than you need. The solution: a beta-blocker that is not inactivated by the liver and provides a more predictable level of beta-blockade, such as atenolol (Tenormin), nadolol (Corgard), betaxolol (Kerlone), bisoprolol (Zebeta), or nebivolol (Bystolic).

SUMMARY

Although beta-blockers lower blood pressure as much as other drugs do, for a lot of people they are the wrong drug, both because they prevent heart attacks and strokes less than other antihypertensive drugs do and because they have more side effects. However, in some people they are exactly the right drug, and the hypertension cannot be controlled without one. If you are suffering side effects from a beta-blocker, there is a lot that can be done to reduce or eliminate them, starting with asking your doctor **if you really need to be on a beta-blocker.** If you feel tired or mentally dull and are taking a beta-blocker, you cannot live the rest of your life without finding out whether the beta-blocker is responsible, and trying one of the options to lessen the problem.

ALPHA-BLOCKERS

Underused, but Fabulous in the Right Patients

Common errors in alpha-blocker use that might be affecting you:

- Your doctor never prescribed one even though your hypertension is uncontrolled.
- You are on a higher dose than you need, increasing the risk of dizziness and fainting.
- You are taking carvedilol (Coreg) or labetalol (Normodyne, Trandate), and it isn't working.

The alpha-blockers (Table 7.1) are both very underused and very misused. Many doctors do not prescribe them because of undeserved negative publicity. Many patients who would respond beautifully are never tried on one. And most doctors who do prescribe them prescribe the excessively high recommended doses, resulting in avoidable side effects.

Alpha-blockers have been engulfed in controversy and have been unfairly maligned. Yes, on average, they lower blood pressure less than other drug classes do. For many, an alpha-blocker is not the right drug. But for many others, they work spectacularly well, including many whose blood pressure might never be controlled without one. In other words, alpha-blockers are fantastic and valuable in the right patient.

In this chapter, I will describe why they are underused, why the negative publicity is unfair and wrong, why they are often prescribed at too high a dose, and who the right patient is.

Table 7.1   The alpha-adrenergic receptor blockers

	Daily doses (mg)		
	Low dose	Medium dose	High dose
Alpha-blockers:			
prazosin (Minipress)	1 twice daily	1–5 twice daily	5–10 twice daily
doxazosin (Cardura)	½ of 1	1–2	4
terazosin (Hytrin)	1	1–2	5–10
Combined alpha/beta-blockers:			
labetalol (Normodyne, Trandate)	100 twice daily	100-300 2–3 times daily	400 3 times daily
carvedilol (Coreg)	3.125 twice daily	6.25–25 twice daily	25 twice daily
carvedilol (Coreg CR)	20 daily	20–80 daily	80 daily

THE PROBLEM WITH ALPHA-BLOCKERS

The alpha-blockers have a major public image problem. It is agreed that they shouldn't be the first drug tried when treating a patient's hypertension, but many doctors are reluctant to add them to other drugs, even in patients with uncontrolled hypertension. Why? Here's the story.

The large ALLHAT trial compared the outcome of treatment of hypertension with each of four drugs: a diuretic (chlorthalidone [Hygroton]), an ACEI (lisinopril [Zestril, Prinivil]), a CCB (amlodipine [Norvasc]), and the alpha-blocker doxazosin [Cardura].[1] Other drugs were then added if needed. The outcome in terms of blood pressure lowering, and prevention of cardiovascular events, such as stroke, heart attack, and heart failure, was then assessed.

Doxazosin, the alpha-blocker, lowered blood pressure 2 mm less than the diuretic did, not a huge difference, but clearly less. The number of strokes and heart attacks was marginally higher, and the incidence of the less common complication of congestive heart failure was doubled. The study organizers concluded that alpha-blockers should not be prescribed as a first-step treatment for hypertension, and dropped doxazosin from the study. These conclusions scared many doctors away from prescribing them, even as add-on drugs.

My experience tells me that an alpha-blocker, given by itself, lowers blood pressure less than other drugs do, in agreement with the ALLHAT findings. I rarely prescribe one by itself as the first drug. But my published research and clinical experience tell me that alpha-blockers are extremely effective when given in the right patient and in combination with certain other drugs, particularly beta-blockers.[2] Alpha-blockers can also be extremely effective when given in combination with an ACEI, ARB, diuretic, or CCB. And in many patients with resistant hypertension, I cannot control the hypertension without prescribing an alpha-blocker.

The accusation that alpha-blockers *cause* heart failure is erroneous. Ironically, carvedilol (Coreg), which is both a beta- and an alpha-blocker, improves heart failure outcomes and is recommended for the treatment of heart failure.[3] Doxazosin did not cause heart failure in ALLHAT; but it is true that it wasn't as effective as the others in preventing it, when used as the first drug.

HOW ALPHA-BLOCKERS WORK

As I discussed in chapter 2, the sympathetic nervous system (SNS) raises blood pressure by stimulating **beta-receptors** and **alpha-receptors** in the heart and arteries. Stimulation of the **beta-receptors** increases the heart rate and force of heart contraction. Beta-blockers block these increases. Stimulation of **alpha-receptors** constricts arteries; alpha-blockers prevent that constriction, allowing the arteries to dilate. **To block SNS-stimulated elevation of blood pressure, the best results are obtained by blocking both the alpha- and beta-receptors, which blocks both the increase in cardiac output and the arterial constriction.**[4]

If the alpha/beta-blocker combination is so effective, should it be used in everyone with hypertension? No. I believe it is most effective in the minority of patients whose hypertension is driven mainly by the SNS, a form of hypertension that is often called "neurogenic hypertension."

What proportion of individuals with hypertension has neurogenic hypertension? My guess is about 15 percent. In chapter 9, I discuss the clues that suggest whether you might have neurogenic hypertension. I believe the most common cause of neurogenic hypertension is "mind/body hypertension," where emotional factors trigger the SNS (chapter 11). Here, my research and clinical experience tell me that the combination of an alpha- and beta-blocker is incredibly effective and should be the treatment of choice, although few doctors prescribe it.

I believe few doctors, in selecting drugs, distinguish between the usual hypertension, which is driven by the kidneys and which responds best to diuretics, CCBs, ACEIs, and ARBs, and neurogenic hypertension, which is driven by the SNS and which I believe responds best to the alpha/

beta-blocker combination. And few doctors are aware of the extraordinary potency of the alpha/beta-blocker combination in mind/body hypertension.

Even though, in the right patient, the alpha/beta combination is incredibly effective, researchers do not study it, partly because of the ALLHAT study and partly because alpha-blockers are now available in generic versions, with no economic incentive for manufacturers to conduct studies. Most research on alpha/beta-blockade focuses on the combination alpha/beta-blockers labetalol (Trandate, Normodyne) and the newer carvedilol (Coreg). Few doctors are aware that these two combination drugs are less effective in lowering blood pressure than when separate pills are prescribed to provide the alpha- and the beta-blockade.[5] And in this era of ACEIs, ARBs, DRIs, and CCBs, neurogenic hypertension is often not on doctors' radarscopes.

WHY DO DOCTORS PRESCRIBE TOO HIGH A DOSE OF DOXAZOSIN?

There is another important, yet rarely mentioned, problem with how alpha-blockers are prescribed: doctors often prescribe too high a dose (table 7.2). Why? Because they are following the manufacturers' recommended doses, which are too high!

The recommended starting dose for doxazosin is 1 mg daily, with titration, if needed, to 2, 4, 8, and even 16 mg daily. These recommendations were based on the manufacturer's studies that assessed doxazosin given by itself. They didn't determine what the dosage should be when it is given in combination with other blood pressure drugs, particularly beta-blockers, even though today doxazosin is rarely prescribed by itself to treat hypertension (it is prescribed by itself to treat prostatism). The dosage recommendations were never changed.

When doxazosin is given in combination with a beta-blocker or an ACEI, I and others have found, and reported, that only 1 or 2 mg is required.[6, 7, 8] Higher doses, which can increase side effects, such as dizziness or fainting, provide minimal benefit. I rarely prescribe more than 2 mg a day.

Table 7.2 Doxazosin: the dosage issue

	Starting dose	Maximum dose
Manufacturer's recommended dosage	1 mg daily	8 or 16 mg
My recommendation	½ or 1 mg daily	2 mg

Doctors almost universally start patients on 1 mg and often have to discontinue the alpha-blocker because of "side effects." Clinical experience has taught me that at least one in four patients responds well to a mere half of the 1-mg pill, and I treat many patients with this low dose. I rarely start a patient of small stature or an elderly patient on a full 1 mg. Yet the use of a half mg is not even mentioned in the medical literature, outside of my own articles.

The risk of dizziness or fainting is greatest after taking the very first dose of doxazosin or any alpha-blocker. That risk can be reduced by starting with a half dose. So even if I think a patient will need 1 mg, I generally recommend taking half of the 1 mg the first day and then increasing to 1 mg. That is also the main reason I prefer doxazosin over another alpha-blocker, terazosin (Hytrin)—doxazosin is a tablet that can be broken in half, unlike terazosin, which is a capsule that cannot broken, eliminating the option of starting with a half dose.

ALPHA-BLOCKERS AND PROSTATISM

Another very important effect of alpha-blockers is that they relax the smooth muscle in the urethra, improving the stream of urine in men with an enlarged prostate. This effect has led to their wide use in men with difficulty urinating due to an enlarged prostate. Currently, alpha-blockers that are more specific for the bladder and urethra, such as tamsulosin (Flomax) and alfuzosin (Uroxatral), which have less impact on blood pressure, are more widely prescribed for prostatism, particularly in men who don't have high blood pressure. But these drugs do lower blood pressure in some patients. In some cases, it is necessary to reduce or eliminate some of the blood pressure medication when starting one of these drugs.

Many urologists prescribe doxazosin at doses of 4 or 8 mg. Some might need that large a dose, but many don't. If you are taking 4 mg or more, and never tried a lower dose, ask your doctor about trying it. If your urinary stream remains stable, you can remain on the lower dose. If not, you can resume the higher dose.

ALPHA-BLOCKERS ON THE MARKET

There are now five alpha-receptor blockers on the market, including three which block only alpha-receptors and two which block both alpha- and beta-receptors (table 7.1). Of the three that block only the alpha-receptors, the most widely used is doxazosin, which I prefer for three reasons: First, its onset of action is more gradual, reducing chances of lightheadedness after the first dose. Second, its duration of action is longer, making its effect more likely to last twenty-four hours. Third, unlike terazosin, it is a breakable pill that allows patients to take half a pill for the first dose.

A new formulation of doxazosin, called doxazosin GITS, is now available in Europe, but not in the United States (as of 2011). It has a more gradual onset and reduces the risk of dizziness or fainting after the first dose. However, even if it is approved for use in the United States, I will never prescribe it, because it is manufactured only at doses of 4 or 8 mg, which is too high for many patients.

The two drugs that block both alpha- and beta-receptors are labetalol (Normodyne, Trandate), and carvedilol (Coreg).[9, 10] I don't often prescribe them for three reasons: First, they don't lower blood pressure as much as a beta-blocker and alpha-blocker given as separate pills. Second, they are metabolized by the liver, resulting in unpredictable blood levels, often too high or too low. Third, I cannot separately increase the alpha-blocking and beta-blocking effects. That is why I prefer prescribing separate pills for the alpha- (doxazosin) and beta-blocking effects. If a patient is taking this combination and the blood pressure is still high and if the heart rate has slowed, indicating beta-blocker effect, I can increase the alpha-blocker dose without having to increase further the beta-blocker effect. If the heart rate has not slowed, I can increase the beta-blocker dose.

For the alpha-blocker, I prefer doxazosin, as discussed above. For the beta-blocker, there are many to choose from (chapter 6), but my favorites are betaxolol (Kerlone), bisoprolol (Zebeta), and nebivolol (Bystolic), whose effectiveness is not affected by metabolism by the liver.

WHAT OTHER DRUGS CAN AN ALPHA-BLOCKER BE COMBINED WITH?

An alpha-blocker can be combined with pretty much any of the other antihypertensive drug classes, including beta-blockers, ACEIs, ARBs, CCBs, and diuretics. But my favorite use is together with a beta-blocker. In chapter 10, I discuss the use of this combination in treating patients with hard-to-control hypertension, where its effect can be dramatic. And in chapter 11, I discuss its use in treating hypertension that is linked to emotional factors, a frequently unrecognized cause of SNS-driven, neurogenic hypertension.

SIDE EFFECTS

The first dose of an alpha-blocker can cause a sharp fall in blood pressure, which can result in dizziness and, rarely, fainting. If you take an alpha-blocker and feel dizzy after the first dose, lie down and eat something salty; it will usually pass.

Although fainting is most likely after the very first dose, it can uncommonly occur after taking the drug for months or even years. A typical scenario: while standing and having a drink (an alcoholic drink lowers blood pressure [chapter 14]). Alpha-blockers also uncommonly cause orthostatic hypotension, meaning a drop in blood pressure upon standing up.

To prevent first-dose dizziness or fainting, I usually recommend taking half of the 1-mg pill for the first dose. In elderly or smaller individuals, or those sensitive to medications, even a quarter pill. By the way, I often prescribe the brand name Cardura for the first dose because it is bigger and easier to break than the generic pill.

Some people feel dizzy even without a fall in blood pressure. I don't understand why this happens; but if needed, I lower the dose or switch to a different drug class.

Finally, alpha-blockers can cause edema, the retention of fluid in the legs. It is not dangerous but can be bothersome. When it occurs, I lower the dose, add a diuretic, or switch to a different drug.

THE PLACE OF ALPHA-BLOCKERS TODAY

Based on studies that show that alpha-blockers lower blood pressure less than other drugs and provide less protection against heart failure, current recommendations do not include an alpha-blocker as a first-step drug for single-drug therapy of hypertension. A diuretic, ACEI, ARB, or CCB is preferred. However, in combination with other drugs such as beta-blockers, CCBs, ACEIs or ARBs, an alpha-blocker is an extremely effective, but underused, add-on drug.

An alpha-blocker is the wrong drug for some and exactly the right drug for others. My studies and clinical experience strongly indicate that their best use is in combination with a beta-blocker in patients with SNS-driven hypertension, such as mind/body hypertension, and in patients with resistant hypertension (chapter 10). I hope more doctors will prescribe them this way.

SUMMARY

Despite negative press, alpha-blockers are very useful, particularly in patients whose hypertension is driven by the SNS. Doxazosin is the most widely used alpha-blocker. I believe the dose range should be ½ to 2 mg, rather than the currently recommended 1 to 16 mg, which is too high. Alpha-blockers are generally not recommended as single-drug therapy for hypertension, but are valuable when combined with a beta-blocker or other drugs.

8

OTHER ANTIHYPERTENSIVE DRUGS

Vasodilators and Drugs Targeting the SNS

VASODILATORS

The vasodilators (table 8.1) do just that—they dilate the arteries. They are not specifically aimed at any of the three mechanisms (sodium/volume, RAS, and SNS). They are options in patients whose blood pressure was not controlled by the drugs that target the three hypertensive mechanisms.

Hydralazine

Hydralazine (Apresoline) is used much less than in the past. The CCBs have largely taken its place. Hydralazine is usually taken twice a day, and is usually prescribed together with both a diuretic, to prevent fluid retention (edema in the legs), and a beta-blocker, to prevent an increase in heart rate. In other words, other drugs are easier to use.

Hydralazine remains an add-on option for resistant hypertension. It is also widely used to treat hypertension in pregnancy, because of its proven safety in pregnant women.

When would I prescribe hydralazine? Mostly for pregnant women and, occasionally, for patients with resistant hypertension.

Table 8.1 The vasodilators, central alpha-agonists, and adrenergic depleters

	Daily doses (mg)		
	Low dose	Medium dose	High dose
Vasodilators			
hydralazine (Apresoline)	10 twice daily	25–100 twice daily	150 twice daily
minoxidil (Loniten)	2.5	5–10	20–40
Central alpha-agonists			
clonidine (Catapres)	0.1 twice to three times daily	0.1–0.4 twice to three times daily	0.6 twice to three times daily
clonidine patch (Catapres patch)	TTS-1, once weekly	TTS-1, 2, or 3, once weekly	TTS-3, 2 patches weekly
guanfacine (Tenex)	½ of 1 mg	1–2	3
methyldopa (Aldomet)	125 twice daily	250–500 twice daily	1,000 twice daily
Adrenergic depleters			
reserpine (Serpasil)	0.1	0.1–0.25	0.5

Minoxidil

Minoxidil (Loniten) is perhaps the strongest arterial dilator available! It is prescribed for severe or very resistant hypertension, but should rarely be used because it is a dangerous drug and tricky to use. It can cause a dangerous degree of fluid retention, even heart failure. It also causes a rapid heart rate. It almost always must be given with a beta-blocker to prevent a rapid heart rate, and a diuretic, sometimes at a massive dose, to prevent fluid retention. Fortunately, few doctors prescribe it. **A doctor who is not very familiar with its use should never prescribe it.**

Minoxidil is actually used widely today, not as an antihypertensive drug, but as a cream applied directly to the scalp to cause hair growth. It is modestly effective.

When would I prescribe minoxidil? Practically never, except as a truly last resort in patients with severe, uncontrollable hypertension.

DRUGS DIRECTED AGAINST THE SNS: CENTRALLY ACTING DRUGS

The Central Alpha-Agonists

The central alpha-agonists lower blood pressure by reducing sympathetic nerve outflow from the brain. They are a very effective option, particularly for patients whose hypertension is driven by the SNS. But in slowing down the SNS, they also slow *you* down. As you might suspect, a drug that acts in the brain often has side effects: commonly, fatigue and sexual dysfunction. They also frequently cause a dry mouth; sounds trivial but it's terrible. Patients say their tongue feels like it is stuck to the roof of their mouth.

Should this limit the use of these drugs? You bet. At an effective dose, fatigue is more the rule than the exception.

The best known of the central alpha-agonists is clonidine (Catapres). Its effect lasts for only eight to twelve hours, and it has to be taken two or three times a day; if you miss a dose or two, your blood pressure can quickly increase. Two other central alpha-agonists have a longer duration of action and steadier blood level: the clonidine patch, which is applied once a week, and guanfacine (Tenex), a pill taken once a day. Unfortunately, the side effects are similar. Also, in many patients, the patch causes a rash.

Most patients are very grateful when I take them off clonidine. A word of caution though: **clonidine should not be stopped suddenly, because that can lead to a withdrawal syndrome, including severe rebound hypertension**. It must be tapered gradually, under a doctor's supervision.

When would I prescribe drugs like these? I prescribe them only when nothing else has worked, or, in the case of methyldopa (Aldomet), in hypertension in pregnancy, where it has a long record of safety. But even here, I usually prefer the alpha/beta-blocker labetalol (Normodyne, Trandate) since it causes less fatigue.

Overall, **I consider the central alpha-agonists the most effective drugs that I try not to use**. However, although most people experience side effects, some don't, so occasionally it's worth a try; but only after other better-tolerated drugs have been tried first.

PUTTING IT ALL TOGETHER

Finding the Drugs and Combinations
That Are Right for You by Aiming
at the Right Mechanism

In the past few chapters, we reviewed the various drug classes. In this chapter we will put it all together. I will describe my strategy for determining which drug or drug combination is right for you. Very simply, **the drug or drug combination that is right for you is the one whose mechanism(s) of action matches the mechanism(s) underlying your hypertension**. Many doctors overlook mechanisms when they prescribe blood pressure drugs. But looking at the three mechanisms enables a very logical and straightforward approach.

A SIMPLIFIED APPROACH FOR PRESCRIBING AND COMBINING DRUGS

The approach is simple: if the mechanism or mechanisms driving your hypertension (table 9.1 and chapter 2) can be identified then the right drug(s) can be selected. For sodium/volume, a diuretic or CCB; for RAS, an ACEI, ARB, or DRI; and for SNS-driven hypertension, a beta-blocker usually together with an alpha-blocker.

Since two of the three mechanisms, **sodium/volume** and the **RAS,** are involved in hypertension in most cases, drug therapy directed at one or both of these two mechanisms will usually bring hypertension under control. In fact, it controls hypertension in 75 percent or more of cases, and will

Table 9.1   The drug classes and the hypertension mechanisms that they target

Mechanism	Preferred drugs
Sodium/volume	Diuretic or CCB
RAS	ACEI, ARB, or DRI
SNS	Beta-blocker often combined with an alpha-blocker

probably control *your* hypertension. But in some patients, treatment must target the third mechanism, the **SNS**, a target that many doctors overlook.

If a single drug controls your hypertension, great. But the odds are about fifty-fifty that more than one mechanism is driving your hypertension and that you will need medication that targets two or sometimes three mechanisms.

The following mechanism-based strategy, which I described in a recent article in the *Journal of Clinical Hypertension*, offers a new approach to treating hypertension that can bring it under control in well over 95 percent of cases. In the next chapter, I present further details for treatment of those with hardest-to-treat hypertension.

Here is the entire strategy in a nutshell:

Table 9.2   A simplified approach for prescribing and combining drugs

1. **If you have ordinary, mild hypertension:**
   - Treatment should start with either a drug that targets sodium/volume (diuretic or CCB) or one that targets the RAS (usually an ACEI or ARB).
   - If it doesn't control your hypertension, target both mechanisms.
2. **If you have more severe hypertension, it is reasonable to start with two drugs, one directed at sodium/volume and the other at the RAS.**
3. **If your blood pressure is not controlled on two drugs, proceed to one or both of the following two options (see chapter 10):**
   - Strengthen the diuretic regimen, usually including addition of a potassium-sparing diuretic.
   - Address the third mechanism, the SNS, usually with an alpha- and beta-blocker, particularly if you have clues that suggest neurogenic hypertension.

WHICH MECHANISM(S) ARE DRIVING YOUR HYPERTENSION?

The obvious question is: which mechanism(s) are driving *your* hypertension, and which medications would be the best fit for treating *your* hypertension? In the next section, I will describe the often overlooked clues that can guide us.

Sodium/Volume

Table 9.3 lists the clues that suggest sodium/volume-mediated hypertension.

Race: In more than half of African-Americans who have hypertension, the mechanism is sodium/volume. A diuretic or CCB will be more effective than an ACEI, ARB, DRI, or beta-blocker. That is why, **in African-Americans, a diuretic or CCB should usually be tried first**.

In whites, all drug classes are equally likely to work. In younger white patients, I would usually try an ACEI, ARB, or CCB first, because they don't have the metabolic side effects that the diuretics and beta-blockers have.

Age: As we age, our kidneys gradually become less efficient in excreting sodium. In many patients, a little assistance by a diuretic is very effective in lowering blood pressure and is a reasonable first choice. Studies show that in patients older than sixty-five, a diuretic or CCB is more likely to work than an ACEI or ARB.[1]

Salt intake: The more salt you consume, the more likely sodium and volume are playing a role in your hypertension and the more likely that you need a diuretic or CCB. If your salt intake is truly low, an ACEI or ARB might work better.

Of course, a high salt intake doesn't raise everybody's blood pressure. If it does, you have what is called **"salt-sensitive" hypertension**, and a diuretic or CCB is likely to work. Salt-sensitivity is determined mostly by genetics.

Among people with hypertension, blood pressure is salt-sensitive in about 25 percent of whites and 50 percent of African-Americans. As we age though, with our kidneys excreting sodium less efficiently, we are increasingly likely to have salt-sensitive hypertension.

You can determine whether or not your hypertension is salt-sensitive by checking your blood pressure at home before and after a few days of

Table 9.3   Five clues that indicate sodium/volume-mediated hypertension

Race
Age
Salt intake
Blood renin level
Evidence of fluid retention

lowering your salt intake. Another way is to have your doctor check your blood renin level, as I discuss next.

Renin: The hormone renin is secreted by the kidneys when our blood volume is low, and triggers the RAS (chapter 2) to retain sodium. When our blood volume is not low, secretion of renin, and activity of the RAS, is suppressed, for example, if we have a high sodium intake.

A low blood renin level, indicative of a suppressed RAS, is telling us that we have ample sodium and volume on board and that a diuretic or CCB will likely lower our blood pressure. It also tells us that an ACEI, ARB, or DRI is less likely to work. A high renin indicates the opposite. The renin test is performed by most commercial laboratories.

Few doctors take advantage of what the renin test can tell us. Ask your doctor about it.

Evidence of fluid retention: If you notice your shoes feeling tighter by the end of the day, and a line of depression in the skin near the top of your socks when you remove them, you are retaining fluid. The retained fluid is called edema. Edema is usually telling us that we have extra volume on board.

If you have edema, a diuretic can kill two birds with one stone: lower the blood pressure and reduce the fluid retention. A CCB would probably also lower your blood pressure but often worsens the edema (chapter 4). If you have edema, a diuretic is a better choice than a CCB.

One caveat: edema doesn't always mean your hypertension is caused by excess volume. In some people edema is caused by "venous insufficiency," a tendency to retain fluid in the legs after prolonged sitting or standing, and has nothing to do with blood volume or blood pressure. Edema can also be due to liver disease. However, usually, edema suggests a volume issue, and the wisdom of prescribing a diuretic.

For Sodium/Volume, which is Preferable: A Diuretic or a CCB?

This is a widely debated question. On average, they lower blood pressure equally, but some people respond better to one than to the other. A recent study, the ACCOMPLISH trial, found that an ACEI/CCB combination prevented heart attack and stroke a little better than an ACEI/diuretic combination, but this result needs to be confirmed in other studies.[2]

Perhaps more important, your doctor should choose between a diuretic or CCB based on which is a better match for you in terms of side effects.

When it is better to avoid a CCB: I would select a diuretic rather than a CCB if you have edema or constipation, either of which can be worsened by a CCB.

When it is better to avoid a diuretic: I would select a CCB rather than a diuretic if you have conditions that can be aggravated by a diuretic:

- Gout, or a high uric acid, which can lead to gout.
- A high risk of developing diabetes (strong family history or slightly elevated blood sugar levels).
- A history of severe allergy to sulfa drugs.

The bottom line: for sodium/volume-mediated hypertension, either a diuretic or a CCB is a reasonable choice as long as it gets the blood pressure down and doesn't leave you with side effects. But aside from that, some people just respond better to one or the other. Go with what works.

Finally, economics shouldn't dictate, but the diuretics are much less expensive.

What If You Are on a Diuretic and Your Hypertension Is Not Controlled? **If sodium/volume is the cause of your hypertension, a diuretic by itself may be enough to control your hypertension.** If your blood pressure does not come under control with a diuretic, there are only three possible explanations:

1) **Sodium/volume *is* the main cause of your hypertension, but the diuretic or dose you are taking is not strong enough**. Your doctor needs to either increase the dose and/or add a potassium-sparing diuretic. I discuss the specifics of strengthening the diuretic in the next chapter.
2) **Your hypertension is driven not only by sodium/volume but also by another mechanism, such as the RAS, and your doctor needs to add a second drug, usually an ACEI or ARB, aimed at the RAS**. Here, if the diuretic lowered your blood pressure somewhat, but not all the way to normal, adding an ACEI or ARB is usually needed to get the job done.
3) **Sodium and volume have nothing to do with your hypertension, and you need a drug or drugs that instead target the RAS and/or the SNS, rather than a diuretic**. If sodium/volume is not a cause of your hypertension and a diuretic didn't lower your blood pressure at all, why continue it? Here your doctor can stop the diuretic and replace it with an ACEI or ARB.

The Renin-Angiotensin System (RAS)

If your hypertension is driven by the RAS rather than by sodium/volume, an ACEI, ARB, beta-blocker, or DRI is more likely to lower your blood pressure than a diuretic or CCB. The obvious question though is, **how can you or your doctor tell if you have RAS-mediated hypertension (table 9.4)?** One clue is demographics: If you are young (under 50) and white, your blood pressure is equally likely to respond to any of the drug classes. But if you are elderly or African-American, your hypertension is more likely to be sodium/volume- rather than RAS-driven, and more likely to respond to a diuretic or CCB than to an ACEI, ARB, or beta-blocker.[3]

Another available, but seldom checked, clue is blood renin activity. If it is high normal or high, a drug that targets the RAS, such as an ACEI or ARB, is more likely to work. A drug that targets the RAS is also more likely to work if your salt intake is truly low.

Another very important clue is how you responded to drugs that were previously tried. If a doctor, in the past, prescribed an ACEI and it had no effect on your blood pressure, your hypertension probably is not driven by the RAS and is more likely to respond to a diuretic than to an ARB.

The Sympathetic Nervous System (SNS)

If your hypertension is driven by the SNS, a form of hypertension called "neurogenic hypertension," I would target neither the RAS (ACEI or ARB), nor sodium/volume (diuretic or CCB). I would instead look to the alpha- and beta-blockers. This is the form of hypertension that they are best suited for.

In chapter 2, I described the two limbs of the SNS, the **adrenal** and the **neural**. Stimulation of the adrenal limb stimulates mainly the beta-receptors, increasing your heart rate and cardiac output. The beta-blockers block this (chapter 6). Stimulation of the neural limb stimulates mainly the alpha-receptors, causing constriction of your arteries. The alpha-blockers block this (chapter 7).

Table 9.4   Clues of RAS-driven hypertension

- Demographics: age and race
- Medium or high renin
- Low-salt diet
- Previous failure to respond to a diuretic

Usually, when the SNS is stimulated, both alpha- and beta-receptors need to be blocked. Many doctors do not realize that blocking just the beta-receptors usually will not do the job. Blocking both, with the underused alpha- and beta-blocker combination, lowers blood pressure considerably.

When treating hypertension, doctors usually think about sodium/volume and the RAS. They often fail to consider SNS-driven hypertension, and **many are unaware of the sometimes dramatic effectiveness of the alpha/beta-blocker combination**, or of the lesser effectiveness of either the alpha- or beta-blocker given alone. This very effective combination can be nearly miraculous in bringing hypertension, and, particularly, resistant hypertension under control, yet is greatly underused.

Drugs like clonidine (Catapres) (chapter 8) are also effective in treating SNS-driven hypertension but frequently cause fatigue, dry mouth, and sexual dysfunction. I consider using them only if alpha/beta-blockade, which is much better tolerated, did not do the job.

One word of caution: even if the SNS is involved in your hypertension, the hypertension can also be partly driven by sodium/volume and RAS, often genetically determined. So your treatment might need to also target these mechanisms.

What Are the Main Causes and Clues of Neurogenic (SNS-Driven) Hypertension?

How can you tell if your hypertension is neurogenic (SNS-driven)? Unfortunately, there is no convenient laboratory method to measure SNS tone. However, there are valuable clues that few doctors pay attention to (table 9.5).

Medical Conditions Associated with Increased SNS Tone   In some cases, there is an obvious medical cause for increased SNS tone, such as in the immediate aftermath of a stroke, alcohol abuse, or sleep apnea (intermittently obstructed breathing at night). Sleep apnea is probably the most common, but mild sleep apnea probably has little impact on blood pressure.

The Pattern of Your Hypertension   In people with neurogenic hypertension, the pattern of the hypertension is often very different from the usual case of hypertension. A very important, yet widely ignored, clue of neurogenic hypertension is the presence of **blood pressure lability**, the tendency of blood pressure to fluctuate considerably. The SNS controls moment-to-moment changes in our blood pressure, and if your blood pressure fluctuates considerably, I would suspect SNS-mediated hypertension. Paroxysmal (episodic) hypertension is a dramatic disorder with sudden

Table 9.5   Clues that suggest neurogenic (SNS-driven) hypertension

1. **Medical conditions associated with increased SNS tone**
   - Immediate aftermath of a stroke
   - Alcohol abuse
   - Sleep apnea
2. **The pattern of your hypertension**
   - Labile blood pressure
   - Paroxysmal (episodic) hypertension
   - Rapid heart rate
   - Hypertension that did not respond to a combination of drugs that target volume and the RAS (e.g., an ACEI/diuretic combination)
   - Unexplained severe hypertension
   - Sudden onset of hypertension
3. **Psychological factors (chapter 11)**
   - History of abuse or trauma
   - Repressive personality type
   - "Wired" personality type

bouts of severe blood pressure elevation. It is almost always a mind/body disorder, as I discuss in chapter 11.

Many people with neurogenic hypertension seem "wired" or anxious, and have a **rapid heart rate,** above 80 beats a minute. Here a beta-blocker, often by itself, can reduce the anxiety, the adrenaline secretion, the heart rate, and with it, the blood pressure. However, if your heart rate is rapid only when you see the doctor, you probably have "white coat hypertension" (chapter 1), which can be considered temporary neurogenic hypertension and might not need treatment.

Another very logical yet widely overlooked clue of SNS-driven hypertension is **"resistant hypertension." If you are taking a drug combination that addresses both sodium/volume and the RAS, such as an ACEI/diuretic combination, and it isn't controlling your hypertension, logic tells us that a different mechanism is likely to be in the mix, with the SNS a prime suspect.**

Another important clue is **severe, unexplained hypertension**. For example, your blood pressure runs 180/120 and there is no obvious reason for it. Here, doctors almost always run tests looking for the uncommon causes of what is called "secondary" hypertension (chapter 12) but find a cause in only about 10 percent of cases. If your hypertension is unusually severe, and you are one of the 90 percent in whom a cause has not been found, the SNS is often the cause.

Another clue is a **sudden rather than gradual onset of hypertension.** This differs from the usual case, where hypertension onset is very gradual.

Psychological Pattern   In most cases of neurogenic hypertension, the cause of the increased SNS tone is considered a mystery. I believe that in most cases psychological factors offer an explanation. However, my research and clinical experience convince me that the mind/body link is very different from what most physicians, patients, and research psychologists think it is. Chapter 11 and my book, *Healing Hypertension: A Revolutionary New Approach* (Wiley, 1999), are devoted to this topic.

The bottom line: in **almost all cases, hypertension can be controlled.** You should not accept the opinion that your hypertension is uncontrollable. And by selecting drugs that match the mechanism of your hypertension, that control can be achieved with the least amount of medication.

SOLVING THE CHALLENGE OF RESISTANT HYPERTENSION

A Simplified, Successful Strategy

COMMON ERRORS IN TREATING RESISTANT HYPERTENSION

- Overtreating due to errors in blood pressure measurement
- Believing mistakenly that a patient's hypertension cannot be controlled
- Failure to refer to a hypertension specialist
- Not prescribing a strong enough diuretic regimen
- Not prescribing an alpha/beta-blocker combination when needed
- Combining drugs that attack the same rather than different mechanisms
- Prescribing minoxidil and clonidine

Many patients are referred to me with "resistant hypertension," technically defined as hypertension uncontrolled on a combination of three or more medications, one of which is a diuretic. In patients with resistant hypertension, the problem is not that the hypertension is uncontrollable or that we lack medication to do the job. The problem, almost always, is that the patient is not on the medications that are right for him or her. In my experience **it is the rare person whose blood pressure cannot be brought under control, as long as we select the right drugs and strategy.** In this chapter, I will focus on a simplified approach for getting hard-to-control hypertension under control.

The problem is that many doctors add drug after drug, without any particular rationale, until either the blood pressure is controlled or side effects have ensued. Often, even with four or five medications, the hypertension is not controlled. And the guidelines for treating resistant hypertension are not that helpful; they advocate adding drugs but offer inadequate guidance as to which drugs.

In a recent paper, I presented a logical and simplified approach for getting the job done.[1] Instead of randomly adding drugs, the approach focuses on just two treatment options, again based on the three mechanisms. The approach, best conveyed as the algorithm shown in figure 10.1, brings resistant hypertension under control 90 percent of the time.[2] There are then other strategies for the few whose hypertension is still not controlled, although frankly, at that point, your doctor should refer you to a hypertension specialist. A list of hypertension specialists, organized geographically, is available online at ash-us.org.

The good news is that you don't necessarily need more medication. As I have emphasized again and again, with the right medication and dosage, your **blood pressure often can be lowered with fewer drugs**. Fortunately, there are many clues to help guide us. But I again caution you not to be your own doctor, but to be a participant with your doctor in the treatment process.

FIRST STEP: MAKE SURE YOU TRULY HAVE RESISTANT HYPERTENSION

I see many patients with supposed resistant hypertension who turn out not to have resistant hypertension at all. In table 10.1, I have listed factors that

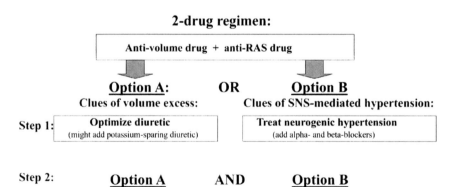

Figure 10.1   Mechanism-based algorithm for treating resistant hypertension
Adapted from Mann SJ. Drug therapy for resistant hypertension: a simplified mechanistic approach. *Journal of Clinical Hypertension* 2011; 13:120–130.

Table 10.1 "Resistant hypertension" that really isn't resistant

- White coat hypertension
- Incorrect measurement of blood pressure in the doctor's office
- Misleading elevation of home blood pressure readings
- Temporary blood pressure elevation
- Isolated diastolic hypertension

frequently create the mistaken impression of resistant hypertension. See if any of these pertain to you before looking at the treatment strategies that follow.

I discuss white coat hypertension, incorrect measurement of the blood pressure at home or in the doctor's office, and temporary blood pressure elevation in chapter 1. It is important to emphasize that if you have well-controlled hypertension, the occasional elevated reading does not mean that your hypertension is "resistant" or out of control.

Isolated diastolic hypertension is elevation of the diastolic pressure with a normal systolic pressure, for example, a reading such as 125/95. If your systolic pressure is normal (i.e., usually below 130 mm) elevation of the diastolic pressure usually does not put you at risk and usually does not require an increase in medication.

BLOOD PRESSURE ELEVATION CAUSED BY OTHER DRUGS

Several widely used drugs can elevate blood pressure and can interfere with achieving a normal blood pressure. The most common offenders are listed in table 10.2 and are discussed in chapter 14. When possible, it is best to stop using them, although if you need them, there are ways they can be prescribed more safely, as I discuss in chapter 14. Only if your hypertension is truly uncontrollable or very severe is it necessary to stop a needed drug. And I don't often encounter that.

Table 10.2 Drugs that elevate blood pressure: the most common offenders

Oral contraceptive pills
Anti-inflammatory drugs
Corticosteroids
Decongestants
Excessive alcohol use

NONPHARMACOLOGIC MEASURES

Even without adjusting medication, there are several important steps you can take. Most important are diet and exercise. Reduction of sodium intake is particularly important, as it increases the effectiveness of most blood pressure drugs. It has been shown to lower blood pressure considerably in patients with resistant hypertension[3] and will likely reduce the amount of medication you need.

A healthy diet, weight loss, exercise, and reduction of excessive drinking add further to blood pressure lowering. Don't underestimate what you can accomplish without pills.

MANAGING TRUE RESISTANT HYPERTENSION

Again I'll get back to the three mechanisms (table 10.3); addressing them is the backbone of treating resistant hypertension logically, successfully, and with the fewest drugs.

As discussed in the previous chapter, in most people, hypertension is driven by one or both of two mechanisms: sodium/volume and the RAS. The combination of a drug that targets sodium/volume (diuretic or CCB) along with one that targets the RAS (usually an ACEI or ARB) will bring hypertension under control in 75 percent of patients. **If you are one of those in whom it doesn't, proceeding to either or both of just two options usually will get your blood pressure under control (table 10.4).**

Table 10.3   The three mechanisms to attack

1. Sodium/volume (volume-dependent hypertension)
2. The renin-angiotensin sytem (RAS) (renin-dependent hypertension)
3. The sympathetic nervous system (SNS) (neurogenic hypertension)

Table 10.4   Treatment of hypertension resistant to drug combinations that target sodium/volume and the RAS

Option 1: Strengthen the diuretic regimen, often by adding a potassium-sparing diuretic, such as spironolactone
Option 2: Add drugs directed at the SNS, usually a combination of an alpha- and beta-blocker

It's that simple! This is the strategy I use to bring hypertension under control in patients who have been treated by doctor after doctor without success, as I recently described.[1] Many physicians fail to take either of these two steps while adding drug after drug, ending up with more and more medication and yet still uncontrolled hypertension. Later in this chapter, I will discuss additional treatment options for the few who don't respond, and in chapter 12, I will discuss secondary hypertension, hypertension with a specific cause that responds to different forms of treatment. Again, though, if your hypertension hasn't responded to the two options, the most appropriate next step would be referral to a hypertension specialist.

The following section presents the details of these two options.

Option 1: Strengthen the Diuretic Regimen

Any discussion of the drug treatment of resistant hypertension must start with the diuretics. The most frequent omission in managing hard-to-control hypertension is failure to prescribe a strong enough diuretic regimen in patients who need one.

Excess sodium/volume, often in patients who are taking the usual dose of a diuretic, is the most frequent cause of resistant hypertension, particularly in this era of high dietary sodium intake. The single most frequent intervention that is needed to bring resistant hypertension under control is strengthening the diuretic regimen.

And the studies concur: **in half of patients with resistant hypertension, the blood pressure comes under control by adjusting the diuretic regimen.**[4, 5] Without strengthening the diuretic regimen, the blood pressure may never come under control, even with four or five drugs. A stronger diuretic regimen not only controls resistant hypertension but also often enables elimination of one or more of the other medications.

If you have ordinary hypertension, a low dose of a diuretic is best because it usually works, and minimizes adverse metabolic effects. And you might not even need a diuretic if your hypertension is not driven by sodium/volume. However, if you have resistant hypertension, particularly if you have a high salt intake or reduced kidney function, the solution will often lie in strengthening the diuretic.

Of course **a high diuretic dose is not for everyone**. If your hypertension is not sodium/volume-driven, a high dose won't help and can do harm. Fortunately, there are clues, usually ignored, that can help identify whether or not you need a stronger diuretic regimen.

Many doctors are afraid to prescribe a strong diuretic regimen when it is needed. A stronger regimen will aggravate a high uric acid level or gout. But if the stronger diuretic is truly needed, the problem is solved by treating the uric acid problem rather than withholding the diuretic dose that is needed.

A stronger diuretic dose can predictably increase the creatinine and blood urea nitrogen (tests of kidney function) a bit, particularly in patients with some degree of kidney disease. This does not mean that the diuretic is damaging the kidneys. It isn't. It does mean that removing the excess fluid, which lowers those numbers, will predictably raise them. When this happens, many doctors lower the diuretic dose, thinking the patient is de-hydrated, and the blood pressure again will be high. Often this is wrong. Eliminating excess volume with a diuretic often requires that these numbers increase a bit (by up to about 25 percent), and unless the increase is excessive, the stronger regimen can usually be safely maintained.

Clues That Suggest That You Need a Stronger Diuretic Regimen
How can you or your doctor tell if you need more than the usual 25 mg of HCTZ? Fortunately there are clues, clues that deserve attention (table 10.5).

You are more likely to need a stronger diuretic regimen if you are big, have a very high sodium intake, or still have edema (fluid retention in your legs). If your blood renin level (chapter 9) is low despite taking a diuretic, it suggests that sodium/volume is still driving your hypertension and that you need a stronger diuretic regimen.

Other standard blood tests can also tell your doctor whether your diuretic dose is enough or not. The blood urea nitrogen (BUN), creatinine, and uric acid levels all increase a bit in response to a diuretic. If they don't budge, it suggests that the dose you are taking might not have done very much, and that a higher dose is worth considering.

Strengthening Your Diuretic Regimen: Your Physician's Choices
There is an art to strengthening the diuretic regimen. Picking the right

Table 10.5   Clues that suggest that you need a stronger diuretic regimen

Your salt intake
Your size
Renin
Edema
Blood tests: blood urea nitrogen (BUN), creatinine, and uric acid
Reduced kidney function

way can help get the best effect with the least harm (table 10.6 and chapter 3).

If you have normal or near normal kidney function, there are three ways to strengthen your diuretic regimen, as listed in table 10.6. Many doctors simply increase the dose of HCTZ from 25 to 50 mg, although this increases the risk of adverse effects, such as a low potassium level (chapter 3). If your doctor chooses to increase the HCTZ dose, I would recommend first trying 37.5 mg (1½ pills) before going up to 50. Also, your doctor must monitor your blood sodium and potassium levels.

A second alternative is switching to the more potent 25 mg of chlorthalidone, which is more or less equivalent to 50 mg of HCTZ (chapter 3). Here again, your doctor should monitor your potassium level and consider adding a potassium-sparing diuretic.

Because of the greater loss of potassium and magnesium with the higher dose of HCTZ or with chlorthalidone, I usually prefer the third option in patients with normal or near-normal kidney function: maintain the 25 mg dose of HCTZ and add a potassium-sparing diuretic (12.5 or 25 mg of spironolactone [Aldactone], 25 or 50 mg eplerenone [Inspra], or 5 or 10 mg of amiloride [Midamor]). This option lowers blood pressure while greatly reducing the risk of potassium or magnesium depletion. If this doesn't control the hypertension, and there are still clues of volume excess (table 10.5), I would increase the dosage of either the HCTZ or the potassium-sparing diuretic, or both, depending on your blood potassium level—if it is low, increase the potassium-sparing diuretic; if high, the thiazide diuretic, or otherwise, either or both. Studies document that spironolactone

Table 10.6   Five ways your doctor can strengthen your diuretic regimen

If you have normal kidney function
  1. Increase HCTZ to 37.5 or 50 mg (consider adding a potassium-sparing diuretic).
  2. Change from 25 mg of HCTZ to 25 mg of the more potent chlorthalidone (consider adding a potassium-sparing diuretic).
  3. Continue HCTZ at 25 mg and add a potassium-sparing diuretic (spironolactone [Aldactone], eplerenone [Inspra], or amiloride [Midamor]). Then increase the dose of either or both drugs if needed.

If you have reduced kidney function
  1. Switch from HCTZ to a loop diuretic, such as furosemide (Lasix) or torsemide (Demadex).

If you have severely reduced kidney function
  1. Prescribe a combination of a loop diuretic along with a thiazide diuretic (HCTZ or metolazone [Zaroxolyn]).

(Aldactone) is very effective in controlling resistant hypertension, but if you develop side effects, your doctor can switch to eplerenone (Inspra) or amiloride (Midamor).

One additional tip: it can take several weeks before the full effect of spironolactone is seen. Your doctor should not jack up the dose or give up on it after only a week or two.

Finally, if you have impaired kidney function, a loop diuretic is usually more effective than a thiazide diuretic. And if you have severely reduced kidney function, the combination of a loop diuretic with a thiazide (HCTZ or metolazone [Zaroxolyn]) may be needed to increase excretion of sodium by the weak kidneys.

Option 2: Add Drugs Directed at the SNS

Many doctors overlook the powerful combination of an alpha- and beta-blocker (chapter 7), even in patients with resistant hypertension. I consider prescribing it in particular in patients with clues that suggest neurogenic (SNS-driven) hypertension (chapter 9, table 9.4).

My experience and research also convince me that much, if not most, of neurogenic hypertension, can be traced to the mind/body connection. I devote the next chapter to this topic.

Although many doctors do prescribe a beta-blocker for resistant hypertension, often it is not effective. If you have neurogenic hypertension, meaning it is driven by the SNS, there are two main reasons why a beta-blocker might fail to lower your blood pressure:

1. You are not "beta-blocked," either because the dose is too low, or the beta-blocker selected is quickly metabolized by the liver (chapter 6). The telltale sign: your heart rate; if it is above 70, you are probably not beta-blocked.
2. It needs to be given in combination with an alpha-blocker (chapter 7). Unfortunately, this combination is woefully underprescribed.

When These Two Options Fail

With either or both of these two options, resistant hypertension should come under control in 90 percent or so of patients. What can your doctor do if both options fail?

Add Other Drugs Your doctor could add drugs, such as spironolactone or a CCB, if you aren't already on them. If they fail, hydralazine (chapter 8), or a drug like clonidine (Catapres) (chapter 8), are options. **I rarely resort to minoxidil** (chapter 8), because it can cause severe and even dangerous fluid retention. However, at this point, I think the best option is referral to a hypertension specialist.

Change the Timing of the Drugs Some drugs last less than twenty-four hours. If your blood pressure is high first thing in the morning and you are taking all your medications in the morning, your doctor can switch one or two of them to the evening, so that their peak effect will occur in the morning.

Consider Secondary Hypertension If your hypertension cannot be controlled, you might have "secondary hypertension" (chapter 12), meaning hypertension that is the result of a specific, sometimes curable cause, such as a narrowing of the artery to the kidney or overproduction of hormones, such as aldosterone or adrenaline by the adrenal gland. One cause, in particular, primary hyperaldosteronism (chapter 12), is much more common among patients with resistant hypertension than we used to think.

In patients with routine hypertension, we don't usually search for those causes, because they are very uncommon, being found in fewer than 1 or 2 percent. However, if you have severe or resistant hypertension, the likelihood is above 10 percent and your doctor should order screening tests. Chapter 12 discusses secondary hypertension.

Invasive Nonpharmacologic Methods You might have read about a couple of new procedures that are being tried: carotid sinus stimulation and renal nerve ablation. Carotid sinus stimulation involves implantation of wires around both carotid arteries in the neck. A current stimulates the carotid nerves and the "baroreceptor reflex," which reduces SNS outflow and blood pressure. This procedure is invasive, leaves scars, and seems barbaric to me. I suspect it will not gain acceptance.

The other and newer procedure is kinder: radiofrequency ablation (destruction) of SNS nerves in the arteries to the kidneys, performed by catheterization through the groin. Early studies suggest it is effective and well tolerated. I am participating in a larger multicenter trial to determine if its efficacy and safety warrant FDA approval. But again, I must emphasize: if the right drugs are used, few people should need these invasive procedures.

SLEEP APNEA

Some patients, particularly obese patients, have "sleep apnea." They experience intermittent obstruction of their upper airway while they sleep. Their breathing literally halts and oxygenation of their blood drops until they finally resume breathing, often with a loud snort. The consequences of repeated deoxygenation of their blood include fatigue, headaches, daytime sleepiness, and hypertension. The diagnosis is made with a sleep study. Treatment, ideally, consists of weight loss. Otherwise, the most widely prescribed treatment, which many find too uncomfortable to use regularly, is a positive pressure mask that improves oxygenation during sleep. Some believe sleep apnea is a cause of resistant hypertension, although studies have not found that wearing the mask lowers blood pressure very much.

Putting it all together, these are the strategies I use in most patients with resistant hypertension. They almost always work. I hope you will discuss these approaches with your physician, and am optimistic that you can achieve a normal blood pressure. If your blood pressure does not come under control, ask to be referred to a hypertension specialist (ash-us.org). You should not give up hope of having a normal blood pressure.

⑪

THE MIND/BODY CONNECTION
AND SELECTION OF THE RIGHT
BLOOD PRESSURE DRUGS

The relationship between psychological factors and hypertension has been an area of considerable interest for decades. There is a widespread belief that there is such a connection, but psychosomatic research has not translated this into definitive evidence or practical consequence. I do believe that there is an important connection but that the link is very different from that which is popularly believed (table 11.1), as I described in my previous book, *Healing Hypertension: A Revolutionary New Approach.*[1] This chapter summarizes my understanding of the mind/body connection with hypertension and its relevance to selecting the right antihypertensive drugs.

It is likely that 30 or 40 percent of hypertension is determined by genetics, and 40 percent or more by lifestyle factors such as diet, weight, salt intake, and lack of exercise. Reflecting this, I believe that **in most people, hypertension is not caused by psychological factors. But I**

Table 11.1   Three core beliefs about the mind/body connection

1. In most cases, hypertension is not driven by psychological factors, but in about 10 to 15 percent, it is.
2. In those whose hypertension is driven by psychological factors, the mind/body link is very different from what most doctors and patients, and you, think it is.
3. Hypertension driven by psychological factors often does not come under control with the usual ACEIs, ARBs, and diuretics. Drugs that address the SNS work much better.

also believe that in about 10 to 15 percent of cases, it is. And when it is, drug treatment is very different than in other cases. That's why it is important to identify whether your hypertension is or isn't related to psychological factors.

Certainly, psychological factors affect hypertension indirectly by interfering with a healthy lifestyle. The absence of will power to watch diet or to exercise clearly has psychological connections, but these indirect effects are not the topic of this chapter.

In this chapter, I want to emphasize two major points:

First, understanding the mind/body connection is not just an exercise in psychology. **Few doctors or researchers realize the relevance of the mind/body connection to selecting the right antihypertensive medication.** Whether psychological factors are, or are not, contributing to your hypertension greatly influences which medications I would prescribe, as I will explain.

Second, I believe **the mind/body connection is very different from what most people think.** In explaining this, I will first describe the usual thinking, which has not helped us understand or treat hypertension, and then describe a different approach, which is a product of my clinical experience, of my studies, and of logic and is strongly supported by psychoanalytic theory. Most important, it is highly relevant to the task of finding the right antihypertensive medication.

THE USUAL PARADIGM, AND WHY IT HAS FAILED TO ADVANCE THE TREATMENT OF HYPERTENSION

The usual paradigm: Hypertension is more likely to occur in people who tend to be tense or angry, or experience considerable day-to-day stress. Techniques that reduce stress can ameliorate or prevent hypertension.

According to this view, if you can learn to handle anger, anxiety, and stress in a better way, you have a better chance of not developing hypertension. This is a neat package, with only one problem. It is wrong (table 11.2). This view dominates psychosomatic research and popular thinking,

Table 11.2   Key questions pertaining to the old paradigm

- Does the tendency to be anxious, angry, or tense cause hypertension?
- Does longstanding stress, such as job stress, cause hypertension?
- Do stress management techniques alleviate or prevent hypertension?

but decades of studies costing billions of dollars have led us nowhere. They have failed to prove that angry or anxious people are at increased risk of developing hypertension. Worse, **that tremendous body of research has had no impact whatsoever on the treatment of hypertension.**

Marie is a worrier. She came to see me because she was very worried about her elevated blood pressure. She also believed that she was causing herself to have hypertension because she worried about everything. And sure enough, her blood pressure was elevated in my office.

Marie is the kind of patient whom many psychosomatic researchers would regard as having a "hypertensive personality." They would teach her relaxation techniques as holistic treatment for her hypertension. If she could learn to relax and to worry less, her hypertension would lessen and she might be able to avoid or get off medication.

I see patients like Marie all the time. The first thing I would tell Marie is that her worrying is not the cause of her hypertension, although it may be the cause of elevation of blood pressure when it is measured (white coat hypertension). The second thing I would tell her is that she might not even have hypertension! And if she does, it is probably because of a genetic predisposition, or weight or diet, and not because of her worrying. Yes, relaxation techniques might help her deal with her worrying, but they have no true impact on hypertension.

The only point in this long-held paradigm that holds up in studies is that when we get angry or anxious, our blood pressure does increase, sometimes substantially. However, this response is temporary. It doesn't persist. If you get angry at your wife, your blood pressure will increase and then come down. Studies indicate that this has little to do with whether or not you will ultimately develop hypertension. **Yes, day-to-day stress does temporarily raise our blood pressure, and yes, stress can make us miserable, but it does not lead to hypertension.**

Does the Tendency to Be Anxious or Angry Cause Hypertension?

Hundreds of studies have examined this question. The results are very inconsistent, and offer support for any and every point of view. Reviews have concluded that there is little if any link.[2, 3] In my own studies, even in people with the most severe hypertension, anger and anxiety scores were no higher than in people with normal blood pressure.[4] My clinical experience is consistent with this.

If anger and anxiety don't lead to hypertension, then what has created the myth that they do, or that tense people are hypertension-prone? One source of this myth is that these emotions clearly do raise our blood pressure in the moment and are often responsible for elevated readings in the doctor's office, often caused by anxiety about the blood pressure measurement. These readings result in overdiagnosis of hypertension and unnecessary treatment in millions of people whose blood pressure, outside the doctor's office, is normal.

The story of a patient of mine dramatically illustrates the absence of long-term effects of emotional distress on blood pressure. Although just an anecdote, it offers a powerful observation that formal studies cannot provide.

I had been following Susan, fifty-six, for borderline hypertension for two years when she informed me that her son, thirty-two, had been diagnosed with an advanced form of cancer and was likely to die. He died a year later. During that year, with constant and severe emotional distress, her blood pressure did not budge one millimeter.

Having interacted with many patients during prolonged emotional crises, I have learned that even severe emotional distress does not lead to sustained blood pressure elevation. This flies in the face of what most people believe, but it is a cornerstone observation that requires us to look for a different paradigm for the mind/body connection in hypertension.

Does Longstanding Stress, Such As Job Stress, Cause Hypertension?

With the many hours we spend at work, if stress caused hypertension, job stress would be high on the list. Clearly job stress can *indirectly* lead to higher blood pressure if it leads to alcohol abuse, overeating, weight gain, or insomnia. But does job stress *directly* cause hypertension? My review of studies on job stress indicates that it does not, with most studies, contrary to expectation, finding either no connection, or very weak and unconvincing evidence.[5] My clinical experience also tells me that it is the rare patient in whom day-to-day stress has a sustained impact on blood pressure.

Do Stress Management Techniques Alleviate or Prevent Hypertension?

Major reviews conclude that they do not.[6] There is no doubt that, in the moment, relaxation techniques, biofeedback, and the relaxation response, as popularized by Herbert Benson, lower blood pressure. But they do not provide a sustained effect. Reflecting this, the use of relaxation techniques to treat hypertension has nearly vanished.

Anxiety-Related Labile Hypertension

One form of hypertension that is clearly related to conscious emotion is *labile hypertension*. Here, patients experience considerable variation in their blood pressure readings, with marked elevations at times of upset or anxiety. Their blood pressure is often normal, but the elevations can be frequent, severe, or both.

Should labile hypertension be treated? We truly don't know. If a patient has frequent and severe elevations, it may be reasonable to treat for three reasons: (1) treatment might prevent complications of hypertension years or decades later, (2) improvement of blood pressure readings will ease the worries of the patient, and (3) the normal readings will also allay the worries of the doctor! However, if the elevations are infrequent, and/or mild, usually there is no need for medication.

In treating this form of mind/body hypertension, I find that drugs directed at the SNS, particularly a beta-blocker or combination of a beta- and alpha-blocker (see chapters 7 and 9), are much more likely to control the hypertension than drug combinations directed at sodium/volume and the RAS. This combination is often incredibly effective. Unfortunately, few physicians employ it, and the hypertension literature barely even broaches the topic of treatment of labile hypertension.

A DIFFERENT UNDERSTANDING OF THE MIND/BODY CONNECTION IN HYPERTENSION

It is not the emotions we feel, but those we have repressed and are unaware of, that lead to hypertension, by causing ongoing stimulation of the sympathetic nervous system (SNS). Antihypertensive drugs that block the effects of the SNS are often effective in controlling this type of hypertension.

This paradigm, virtually the opposite of the other, focuses on the tendency to repress rather than feel painful emotion. It is not the day-to-day distress that we feel that causes hypertension. It is instead what we have repressed and don't feel that persists within us and, even without our awareness of it, can produce longstanding stimulation of the SNS and blood pressure elevation.

The emotions we repress are often much more powerful and painful than the day-to-day feelings we consciously experience. These emotions persist within us, even though we are not conscious of them and are not aware that we are repressing them. They don't come and leave. They stay but are hidden from our awareness. In my experience, people who regularly experience emotional distress are less likely to develop hypertension than people who repress emotion and almost never experience emotional distress.

The following example dramatically illustrates the link I have repeatedly observed between repressed emotion and hypertension.

Jim, forty-four, was a tall, slim, very successful and recently married African-American man who had recently been diagnosed with incurable metastatic cancer. He was referred to me after developing moderately severe hypertension, even though he was eating little and had lost 30 pounds, which if anything should have lowered his blood pressure.

With no other apparent cause, it would seem logical to blame his hypertension on severe distress concerning his diagnosis and poor prognosis. However, and I will never forget his answer, when I asked him if he was very upset, he responded seriously and not sarcastically, "No, I'm not upset. Why should I be upset?" He truly did not feel upset!

This is a classic example of denial of emotions that might be too painful to bear consciously. If Jim had been distraught, everyone would have readily attributed his hypertension to the distress. The usual thinking, however, does not make sense in this case; the new paradigm does. In fact, no other explanation, medical or psychological, can make sense of this case (tests for causes of secondary hypertension were negative). As I found out, in many cases, **it is the patient's *story* rather than the *emotions* he or she describes that often make sense of neurogenic, SNS-mediated hypertension.**

I want to emphasize that repressing emotions at times of overwhelming stress is not psychopathology. It is an emotional defense that serves us, helping us to cope with overwhelming emotion, such as that which follows severe emotional trauma. It keeps us from being wrecked by emotional distress that may exceed our coping capacity. Yes, I believe repression can lead to hypertension and probably to other psychosomatic conditions as well, but it can save us from psychological ruin. Our ability to repress emotion often is a true blessing, but it does contribute to hypertension, sometimes severe hypertension.

REPRESSION

We are fortunate in having at our disposal both *conscious* and *unconscious* defenses to deal with extremely painful emotion. We all make *conscious* efforts to avoid emotions that are painful to us, for example by keeping busy. Repression is very different. It is an *unconscious* defense that, without our even knowing it and without any conscious effort on our part, protects us from feeling deeply painful emotions. When we are repressing painful emotions, we are usually unaware that we are doing so. It is as if we are on autopilot—we just don't feel the emotional pain, essentially a gift from our unconscious defenses.

An example that illustrates conscious and unconscious defenses is the process of grieving. We could not function during the grieving process if we were overwhelmed by the pain all day every day. We use our defenses, both conscious and unconscious, to shield us from the pain. Sometimes we repress the pain and, seemingly without effort, don't feel it. We even seem surprised that we feel okay, almost as if nothing had happened. Even though we clearly *know* that we have been deeply wounded, we don't *feel* it. Other times we feel the pain, and make a conscious effort to keep it out of mind by focusing on other things. And, of course, there are other times when the pain sears us, when we actually are doing the work of healing by feeling the pain until it eventually begins to ease and becomes more tolerable. We are psychologically healthiest when we can use conscious and unconscious defenses to tamp down emotions that are too much for us, enabling us to encounter these emotions at a pace we can handle and deal with, and to ultimately heal. And in the case of truly overwhelming trauma, we are probably better off never facing those emotions.

I have seen many patients who were survivors of severe abuse or trauma. Some experienced severely painful emotion and gradually healed, leaving a residue of painful but tolerable feelings that come up from time to time. Others though, who continued to be affected by deeply painful emotions, suffered psychologically the rest of their lives, with manifestations such as chronic anxiety, depression, or post-traumatic stress disorder.

Still others coped by repressing, and escaped such consequences. They may have felt deep pain at the time, perhaps for days or weeks or longer, but then ultimately repressed. They remember the story of their trauma but suffer no conscious lingering pain. Although repression can lead ultimately to consequences such as hypertension, at least the hypertension can be controlled with the right medication, and I would think that is preferable to lifelong emotional torment.

Repression That Leads to Hypertension

We all repress. Even without trauma, we are bombarded with so much that it would be hard to live our lives without repressing some of it. We can't react to everything. In my experience, though, repression that leads to hypertension is different.

In my experience, two patterns of repression seem to be associated with the development of hypertension (table 11.3):

1. Repression related to severe abuse or trauma: I have seen many patients who have repressed emotion related to prior severe abuse or trauma, from as long ago as childhood. Few consider its role in current illness because it happened so long ago and also because they don't experience emotional distress related to it.

Those who have repressed overwhelming trauma-related emotions often report that they do not experience any lingering psychological effects. They insist that they put the trauma behind them and moved on, which is in fact what they did. They are truly different from trauma survivors who readily acknowledge lingering emotional pain.

A history of trauma is not rare. Over 20 percent of people report a history of severe abuse or trauma, particularly during childhood.[7] Sadly, **research psychologists largely ignore what I suspect is an important link between childhood experience and adult hypertension**, focusing instead on more mundane day-to-day anger and anxiety.

When a physician sees such a trauma survivor whose hypertension is related to the trauma, he will not suspect a mind/body link both because the trauma is usually decades old and because the patient neither mentions the old trauma nor reports any emotional distress related to it. Again, the clue lies not in the *emotional distress* patients report but in their *story*.

2. Repression as a day-to-day coping style: I see many patients who don't have a past history of abuse or trauma but who are repressors. We all know people who are very even-keeled, who are always "up," who rarely get upset, even about the major stuff that gets to most of us.

Table 11.3   Clues that suggest repression-linked hypertension

1. A history of severe abuse or trauma, particularly during childhood, particularly with the belief that the trauma has had no lingering effects
2. A very even-keeled personality, a person who is never "down"

In my experience, this tendency is associated with hypertension. This may seem counterintuitive, but it is what I have observed repeatedly and consistently. It is saying that someone who never feels down or depressed, no matter what is going on in his or her life, is more prone to develop hypertension than someone who does feel a bit depressed from time to time.

When I ask a patient if he ever feels down or depressed, a repressor will respond "never," no matter what problems he has had to endure. He is not holding in feelings of depression, anxiety, or anger. He truly doesn't feel them.

These observations are supported by the results of many studies. In his meta-analysis of psychological studies, Randall Jorgensen found emotional defensiveness, the tendency to be unaware of emotions, to be the psychological measure most powerfully linked to hypertension.[2] I also found this to be true, particularly in people with severe hypertension.[4]

What underlies a person's tendency to handle stress this way? Some people are just born that way. Others might have grown up in a family that did not discuss or share feelings or emotional pain, or had a macho philosophy about not yielding to emotional pain. Growing up with no one available for emotional support, they learned, by necessity, to numb themselves, to not feel. Yes, a person can be emotionally alone even if surrounded by a large family.

Does this mean that being a calm person per se puts you at risk of developing hypertension? No. Some people are calm and handle day-to-day stress calmly. They "don't sweat the small stuff." That's great. However, when we don't sweat the big stuff either, that is when the sympathetic nervous system (SNS) is activated.

Do All Repressors Develop Hypertension?

Certainly not. Many repressors have a normal blood pressure. But the likelihood of developing hypertension, and the severity of the hypertension that develops, is greater. And of course hypertension is most likely to develop in those who are already hypertension-prone from factors such as genetics (family history of hypertension) and obesity.

I also believe that individuals with a repressive coping style are more likely to develop hypertension if they have encountered a great deal of severe life stress. Even if you are a repressor, if you have been lucky enough to live an easy life, you are less likely to develop hypertension than if you have lived a difficult life.

EPISODIC (PAROXYSMAL) HYPERTENSION, AKA "PSEUDOPHEOCHROMOCYTOMA"

I have pioneered the description of this form of hypertension, which is almost always a result of the mind/body connection and is almost always linked to repressed emotion.[8, 9] Patients with this form of hypertension experience sudden and recurrent episodes of blood pressure elevation that in many cases is quite severe, accompanied by severe physical symptoms such as headache, shortness of breath, weakness, lightheadedness, or sweating. The episodes typically occur "out of the blue," bearing no relationship to perceived stress. They can last minutes to hours and are often followed by exhaustion. They can occur daily or only once every few days, weeks, or months. In between episodes, the blood pressure can be normal or near normal.

The episodes feel horrible; patients may feel like they are going to die or have a stroke. Many live in fear of the next attack and are afraid to go about their normal activities. Many have to stop working.

Paroxysmal hypertension always arouses the physician's suspicion of a tumor of the adrenal gland, called a pheochromocytoma (or pheo for short), that secretes adrenaline and/or noradrenaline. But a pheo is found in only 1 to 2 percent of cases. The other 98 percent had been a longstanding medical mystery, but its link to repressed emotion, related to either past trauma or a repressive coping style, has made sense of it and led to treatment options that are usually effective.[9] Unfortunately, few doctors are aware of this understanding, and nearly all patients go from doctor to doctor without uncovering the cause or receiving the appropriate treatment.

Few doctors realize that "paroxysmal hypertension" is very different from "labile hypertension." With labile hypertension, blood pressure swings usually accompany emotional upset; patients are aware that they are upset and that the increase in blood pressure is a result of that distress. The blood pressure swings are clearly caused by SNS reaction to emotions in the moment. With paroxysmal hypertension, the blood pressure swings come seemingly out of nowhere without any relationship to current stress or distress.

The Mind/Body Connection and Drug Therapy of Hypertension

It is well established that the SNS is responsible for the transient increases in blood pressure that we experience when we feel emotions such as anger or anxiety. It makes sense that the SNS also mediates the effects on blood pressure of repressed emotions, which are more powerful than the emotions we feel and are more long-lived.

That is why hypertension that is linked to psychological factors differs from the usual case of hypertension. Getting back to the three basic mechanisms, it is driven by the SNS rather than by sodium/volume and/ or the RAS. And that is why it requires different medication, specifically, medications directed at the SNS. My experience and research indicate strongly that mind/body hypertension often cannot be controlled with the usual drug therapy that is directed at sodium/volume and the RAS, and requires a different set of drugs. That is also why I consider the possibility of SNS-mediated hypertension in patients whose hypertension is resistant to a combination of anti-volume and anti-RAS drugs. However, virtually no research has looked at this difference in selecting drug therapy, probably because medical researchers are not interested in psychology, and research psychologists are not interested in antihypertensive medications.

Drug Therapy of Psychologically Linked Hypertension

As I described in chapter 2, stimulation of the SNS usually stimulates both the **adrenal limb,** with adrenaline stimulating mostly the beta-adrenergic receptors, resulting in an increase in heart rate and cardiac output, and the **neural limb,** with noradrenaline stimulating mostly the alpha-adrenergic receptors, resulting in increased arterial constriction. Together these effects increase blood pressure. Alpha- and beta-blockers, given in combination, are very effective in treating SNS-driven (neurogenic) hypertension.[10, 11] Other drugs, such as clonidine, also work (chapter 8), but side effects such as fatigue are a problem in most patients.

In my experience, hypertension attributable to the mind/body connection often is not controlled by the usual combination of drugs directed at sodium/volume (diuretic or CCB) and the RAS (ACEI or ARB) but responds, often dramatically, to the alpha- and beta-blocker combination (chapter 7). I have also observed this in my research. For example, I observed that an ACEI or diuretic controlled hypertension in only 25 percent of patients who reported a history of childhood abuse or trauma, but in 75 percent of patients without such a history![12] And the alpha/ beta-blocker combination worked very well in the trauma survivors. I also find consistently, although I have not performed a formal study, that in patients with labile hypertension, an alpha/beta-blocker combination is much more effective than combinations of diuretics, CCBs, ACEIs, and ARBs. Unfortunately, the alpha-blockers were out of favor for the past decade and few doctors recognize the potency of the alpha/beta-blocker combination, particularly in patients like John.

John, thirty-five, developed severe hypertension shortly after being diagnosed with AIDS. The combination of an ACEI and a diuretic didn't touch his blood pressure, which remained at 180/120. His doctor considered the possibility, in line with the old paradigm that severe emotional distress related to the diagnosis was causing the hypertension, but rejected that explanation because John did not seem at all upset. He seemed really "cool" about it.

The new paradigm tells me exactly the opposite: the absence of distress where severe distress would have been expected was the clue that John was repressing highly threatening emotion, and that his hypertension *was* psychologically mediated. Treatment with an alpha/beta-blocker combination promptly normalized his blood pressure.

Avoid Excessive Doses of Drugs That Are Unlikely to Work

One warning: when a diuretic/ACEI combination does not control hypertension, it is common practice to increase the dosage of one or both drugs. Often a higher dose is necessary, particularly that of the diuretic. But if your hypertension is neurogenic (SNS-driven), the alpha/beta combination is much more likely to do the job, while a high dose of the diuretic is not needed and can confer harm. This is why recognizing when emotional factors are integral to the hypertension, and when they are not, is so important in getting on the right drugs and avoiding excessive doses of drugs that are unlikely to control your hypertension.

Management of Episodic (Paroxysmal) Hypertension (Pseudopheochromocytoma)

Paroxysmal hypertension is a dramatic, hard-to-control, and disabling form of neurogenic hypertension and is widely mistreated. Here are two typical cases:

Frank, sixty-five, ran a corporation, until hypertensive episodes disabled him. The attacks would occur out of the blue about once a week. He would suddenly develop a severe headache and feel flush, and his blood pressure would soar to 200/120. Doctors suspected a pheo, but tests had found no abnormality.

Frank was a doer, not a feeler. He was never anxious or depressed. He was a repressor. He described an auto accident which left his son permanently paraplegic. I said to him, "I'll bet you never cried." And he replied, "You're goddamned right."

Sarah was a Holocaust survivor. She was fine until she turned seventy and then began to experience sudden and disabling hypertensive attacks. Tests for a pheo were negative. She insisted that the Holocaust had had no lingering emotional impact.

To date, the explanation and treatment approach for paroxysmal hypertension that I offer in this chapter is the only approach in the medical literature that offers a path to successful treatment. Even though it is successful in most cases, few doctors employ this approach, because neither the concept of repressed emotion, nor the thought of using an antidepressant to treat a hypertensive disorder, is widely understood or accepted.

I have reported the following principles as cornerstones of treating paroxysmal hypertension:[8, 9]

1. In those able to acknowledge the underlying repressed emotions, the episodes might cease even without medication. In many cases though, the repressed emotions are too overwhelming to go back to.
2. Rapid-acting blood pressure medication that targets the SNS (such as the alpha/beta-blocker labetalol, given intravenously, or clonidine, given orally) and/or a rapid-acting benzodiazepine tranquilizer, such as alprazolam (Xanax), are useful in lowering blood pressure during attacks.
3. Taking a daily dose of an alpha/beta-blocker may or may not prevent future attacks but usually reduces the severity of the blood pressure elevation.
4. Reassurance goes a very long way: reassurance that the condition is not a mystery, reassurance that attacks are extremely unlikely to cause a sudden stroke or death, and reassurance that a return to a normal life is possible and likely.
4. In those in whom frequent severe attacks continue to occur, and to interfere with day-to-day life, an antidepressant is usually dramatically effective, and, within two weeks, usually eliminates hypertensive attacks and restores a normal life.

I believe the antidepressant works by strengthening the barrier to awareness of threatening, overwhelming emotions. It is an example *par excellence* of mind/body hypertension, and the best example of a medical disorder that can be successfully treated with a drug used for psychological rather than medical diagnoses. The effectiveness of an antidepressant in this hypertensive disorder is perhaps the most blatant evidence that the mind can be involved in hypertension and that the mind must be considered in assessing patients with difficult-to-control hypertension. It also raises the question of the role of repressed emotion in other medical illnesses whose origin is a mystery, such as asthma, migraine, inflammatory bowel disease, fibromyalgia, and others, in which a mind/body connection has been suspected but never clarified.

Is There a Role for Psychotherapy?

As I have discussed, relaxation techniques can relieve stress in the moment but do little for hypertension. Would psychotherapy help? If I am correct in my understanding, the surprising answer is usually, but not always, no! Here's why.

When I see patients whose hypertension is linked to repression of emotions related to prior abuse or trauma, and discuss that link with them, some get the connection and experience an abrupt, and healing, shift in awareness concerning their past. The hypertension sometimes melts away with this shift, even without psychotherapy. Psychotherapy though can be helpful in dealing with the emotions that come up.

However, I believe that for most patients, psychotherapy to explore overwhelming but repressed emotions is not likely to achieve anything. They are not suffering emotional distress, do not feel any need for psychotherapy, and are not interested in it. Many clearly do not want to go anywhere near those emotions, and, in fact, exploring repressed trauma-related emotions might be the wrong thing for them to do. The therapy would be unlikely to crack the repression, and if it did, it could do harm.

Patients who come to see me for their hypertension didn't come to me to explore old trauma; they came seeking to bring their hypertension under control. Although I am an advocate of recognizing the mind/body relationship in hypertension, I would argue against coercing reluctant patients, who survived well by repressing, to seek psychotherapy and attack that repression. It is wise to honor a patient's preference to not explore the past.

In other words, the catch-22 of psychotherapy in hypertension is that the more aware a patient is of emotional distress and the more willing the patient is to pursue psychotherapy, the less likely it is that psychological issues are the cause of that individual's hypertension! And the more a trauma survivor insists that the past has had no lingering impact, indicating repression, the more likely it is that the hypertension *is* related to it, but the less likely that he or she will be amenable to, or helped by, psychotherapy.

SUMMARY

If your hypertension is strictly a matter of genetics and lifestyle, and has nothing to do with psychological factors, I would usually select drugs from among the diuretics, CCBs, ACEIs, and ARBs. But in the 15 percent or so whose hypertension is linked to the "mind/body" connection, and is driven by the brain and the SNS rather than by the kidneys, drug treatment is very different. An alpha/beta-blocker combination is much more likely to lower blood pressure. Few doctors realize the nature of the mind/body connection and the need to treat with drugs that address the SNS rather than the other drugs.

It is my belief that the mind/body connection is not involved in the usual case of mild hypertension that responds to an anti-volume drug, or an anti-RAS drug, or a combination of the two. It is more likely to be involved in patients with severe or resistant hypertension, and nearly certain to be involved in patients with labile or paroxysmal hypertension. It is in them that treatment directed at the SNS should be kept in mind.

Of course, in people with mind/body hypertension, genetic and/or lifestyle factors can also be involved. In them, the best treatment may be an alpha/beta-blocker combination along with a diuretic and/or ACEI, and, of course, a healthy lifestyle.

⑫

SECONDARY HYPERTENSION

This book focuses on the 95 percent of people considered to have "essential hypertension," meaning there is no specific identifiable cause beyond the genetic, lifestyle, and mind/body factors that increase the likelihood of developing hypertension. There is no specific cure, although the hypertension can usually be controlled by a healthier lifestyle and/or lifelong medication.

But in up to 5 percent of cases, there is a specific cause. Here hypertension is regarded as "secondary hypertension," meaning the hypertension is secondary to a specific cause. Treatment usually differs from that of ordinary essential hypertension, and with the right treatment, the amount of medication often can be reduced. In some cases, the hypertension can even be cured. In other words, if you have secondary hypertension, it's worth knowing it. Although the diagnosis and management of secondary hypertension is not the focus of this book, in this chapter I will provide a brief summary of the main causes of secondary hypertension and their treatment (table 12.1).

Should your doctor perform screening tests to see if you have secondary hypertension? For ordinary mild hypertension, no. The odds are probably less than one in a hundred of finding a cause. But if there are clues that suggest secondary hypertension (table 12.2), there is a 10 percent likelihood and it is worth looking for. In general, if it just doesn't make sense that you have hypertension, or severe hypertension, think of secondary hypertension.

Table 12.1   Common causes of secondary hypertension

1. Primary hyperaldosteronism (excess production of aldosterone)
2. Renovascular hypertension (blockage in the artery to the kidney)
3. Kidney diseases
4. Medications (birth control pill, anti-inflammatory drugs, others) (chapter 14)
5. Cushing's syndrome
6. Pheochromocytoma
7. Narrowing (coarctation) of the aorta

CLUES THAT SUGGEST SECONDARY HYPERTENSION

Some clues suggest secondary hypertension but don't point to a specific cause. Other clues point at a specific cause.

General Clues

A clue that should always trigger some suspicion is severe hypertension, with readings often above 180/110, and especially if readings are much higher. If you are someone who "shouldn't" have hypertension, that too is a clue. If you are young and thin, exercise regularly, and have a low salt diet, and no one in your family had hypertension, even if your hypertension is not severe, it makes no sense that you have hypertension. A search

Table 12.2   Clues that suggest that you might have secondary hypertension

General clues

- Severe hypertension
- Hypertension in someone who "shouldn't" have hypertension
- Hypertension that doesn't respond to the usual medication
- Sudden onset
- Young age at onset of severe hypertension

Specific clues

- Low potassium level
- Bruit (murmur) heard in the abdomen in the region of the artery to the kidney
- Lower blood pressure in the legs than in the arms
- Episodic hypertension
- Reduced kidney function
- Protein in the urine

for a cause is justified. If you weigh 250 pounds, eat a ton of salt, and don't exercise, it isn't.

Essential hypertension usually develops gradually, usually starts in our thirties, forties, and fifties, and usually responds to standard medication. If your blood pressure was 120/80 a year ago and is 170/110 now, if you developed marked hypertension in your teens or twenties, or if the usual medication did not control your blood pressure, it would raise suspicion.

Specific Clues

If your blood potassium level is low, particularly if you are not on a diuretic that lowers the potassium level, it is a strong sign of excessive circulating aldosterone and possible primary hyperaldosteronism (see below). A bruit (murmur) heard in the abdomen in the region of the artery to the kidney suggests a narrowing of the artery to the kidney. If you are young and the blood pressure in your legs is lower than the blood pressure in your arms, it suggests a narrowing of your aorta (the body's largest artery that carries blood from the heart down to the lower abdomen), usually a congenital condition called a coarctation of the aorta. However, if you are older, lower blood pressure in the legs is usually due to atherosclerosis in the arteries in your legs rather than a coarctation of the aorta.

CAUSES OF SECONDARY HYPERTENSION

Primary Hyperaldosteronism

Among patients with resistant hypertension, primary hyperaldosteronism is the cause in as many as 10 to 20 percent, much more common than most doctors realize.[1] Even today, many physicians fail to consider and look for it and the path to treatment or even cure that it offers.

The cause is overproduction of the hormone aldosterone by the adrenal gland (chapter 2), which results in retention of sodium and excretion of potassium by the kidneys. The result: elevation of blood pressure and a low blood potassium level. Retention of sodium and volume suppresses secretion of renin (chapter 2), resulting in **the classic triad of primary hyperaldosteronism: low levels of blood potassium and renin, with a high aldosterone level (table 12.3).** The excessive aldosterone secretion usually originates either from overgrowth in both adrenal glands or from an aldosterone-secreting nodule (adenoma) in one gland.

Table 12.3 The three classic findings in patients with hypertension caused by primary hyperaldosteronism

1. Low potassium level
2. High aldosterone level
3. Low renin level

If you have severe or resistant hypertension, and a low potassium level that is not caused by a diuretic, you probably have primary hyperaldosteronism and bells should go off in your doctor's head. The low potassium level is virtually screaming out the diagnosis.

Diagnosis Screening for the disorder is simple: **a blood sample to check the potassium, renin, and aldosterone levels**. If the potassium and renin levels are low and the aldosterone level is high, the diagnosis is probable.

What many doctors don't realize though is that the potassium level can be normal, making the diagnosis far less obvious. That's why, even if your potassium level is normal, your doctor should screen for hyperaldosteronism if you have unexplained severe or resistant hypertension.

If the tests suggest primary hyperaldosteronism, the next task is to determine whether the aldosterone is being secreted by the left, right, or both adrenal glands. If it is coming from just one gland, there is a choice of treatment: a potassium-sparing diuretic (chapter 3) to control the condition by blocking the effects of aldosterone, or laparoscopic surgery to remove the gland (in some cases the adenoma can be removed without removal of the entire gland), which in some cases can cure the hypertension. If the oversecretion is coming from both glands, pills are the only option; it would be harmful to remove both glands.

The two main tests used to determine whether excessive aldosterone secretion is coming from one or both glands are: (1) a **scan of the adrenal glands** (CT scan or MRI) to detect whether one or both glands are abnormal and (2) **adrenal vein sampling**, done by catheterization, to determine whether it is the left, right, or both adrenal glands that are secreting the aldosterone.

Renovascular Hypertension

Renovascular hypertension is caused by narrowing or complete blockage of the artery supplying blood to a kidney. The kidney, sensing that it is not getting enough blood, secretes renin to raise blood pressure in an attempt to increase its blood flow. Getting back to the three hypertension mechanisms, the RAS (renin-angiotensin system) is the mechanism driving renovascular hypertension.

Renovascular hypertension, which is responsible for hypertension in about 1 or 2 percent of people with hypertension, tends to happen in two groups:

- *Older* individuals with atherosclerosis of their arteries usually caused by decades of smoking and/or elevated cholesterol levels.
- *Younger* individuals, mostly women, with arteries scarred and narrowed by *fibromuscular dysplasia*, an inflammatory process of unknown cause. I would consider fibromuscular dysplasia in young patients with unexplained or severe hypertension.

The gold standard diagnostic test for renovascular hypertension is the renal arteriogram, which involves inserting a catheter into the femoral artery in the groin, threading it up the aorta to the arteries that supply the kidneys, and injecting dye to visualize them. The test is expensive, is invasive, and requires injection of dye, although the amount of dye is small and unlikely to be toxic to the kidneys. If a narrowing in the artery is seen, it can be dilated and stented. The dye however can be toxic to the kidneys in patients with reduced kidney function, and minimizing the amount of dye used is crucial.

Fortunately, there are less invasive screening tests that when negative, obviate the need for the invasive arteriogram. The two most widely used tests are the sonogram (ultrasound) and the MRA.

Sonography of the kidney with Doppler examination of the renal arteries is noninvasive and inexpensive, but its accuracy depends on the skill of the technician.

MRA (Magnetic Resonance Angiography) provides a noninvasive angiogram. It uses a different dye, gadolinium, which is not toxic, except uncommonly in patients with reduced kidney function.

Other less invasive options include the CT angiogram and the renal scan. A **CT angiogram** obtains images using dye that is injected into a vein in the arm. It is less accurate than an angiogram and involves a larger dose of dye, which can be toxic to the kidneys in patients with reduced kidney function. A **renal scan** visualizes each kidney's uptake, using a radioactive tracer. Its use has declined in recent years

Renal artery stenosis can usually be repaired by balloon dilation with or without placement of a stent. Less commonly it is repaired surgically. The alternative of treatment with antihypertensive medication is an option and should usually include an ACEI or ARB to antagonize the RAS. However, without dilating the artery, the kidney may gradually lose its function.

Whether angioplasty with stenting is preferable to the noninvasive alternative of blood pressure control with medication is controversial. A few recent large trials concluded that it provides no benefit, but prior studies and clinical experience indicate with certainty that it does benefit some patients. As I wrote in a recent editorial, some patients clearly do benefit from the procedure, but it is important to avoid the procedure in those who are least likely to benefit and/or most likely to suffer adverse effects.[2]

In general, in younger patients, I recommend angioplasty to avoid permanent loss of function of the kidney. In a very old patient, I would continue medication and avoid the risks of angioplasty unless the hypertension cannot be controlled or the kidney function is deteriorating.

Other Kidney Diseases

Almost any disease that reduces kidney function can cause hypertension. Either or both of two of the mechanisms we have discussed underlie blood pressure elevation in most cases: sodium/volume and the RAS. With kidney disease, hypertension can be caused by reduction in the amount of sodium that the kidneys can excrete and/or by an increase in the kidneys' secretion of the hormone renin, which activates the RAS (chapter 2). In some cases, kidney disease can be suspected by the presence of protein or blood in the urine. In other cases, there is no abnormality whatsoever on urinalysis, but blood tests (elevation of creatinine or blood urea nitrogen [BUN]) indicate reduced kidney function.

Treatment with a diuretic to increase sodium excretion, usually with an ACEI or ARB to antagonize the RAS, can usually control the hypertension. **The most common error that physicians make in treating hypertension caused by kidney disease is prescribing an insufficient dose of the diuretic.** The more advanced the reduction in kidney function, the stronger the diuretic regimen needed (chapter 10). Also, if your kidney disease is advanced, your doctor should probably prescribe a loop diuretic rather than a thiazide diuretic (chapters 3 and 10). If you have very advanced kidney disease, the powerful combination of a loop diuretic and a thiazide diuretic may be needed. A nephrologist should be consulted to determine the cause of the kidney disease and whether there is any treatment to halt the kidney damage.

If you have kidney disease, maintaining a normal blood pressure is by far the most important factor in preventing or delaying progression to kidney failure and dialysis. If you have kidney disease and your blood pressure is not under control, get to a specialist (nephrologist or hypertensionist) as soon as possible.

Cushing's Syndrome

Cushing's syndrome is an uncommon condition caused by excessive levels of cortisol, a hormone secreted by the adrenal gland. An excess of this hormone causes a constellation of abnormalities, including blood pressure elevation and weight gain, particularly in the trunk, sometimes accompanied by dramatic change in facial appearance and often by development of diabetes.

The cause can be a tumor in the adrenal gland, or overstimulation of the adrenal gland by the pituitary gland or by corticosteroid pills, such as prednisone, that are given to treat various health disorders. Testing involves a blood test or twenty-four-hour urine collection to measure the hormone cortisol.

If you have an excess of this hormone, your treatment should be managed by an endocrinologist.

Pheochromocytoma

Pheochromocytoma (pheo for short) is a rare tumor that usually arises in the adrenal gland and secretes the hormones adrenaline and/or noradrenaline. It occurs in perhaps 1 in 300,000 people with hypertension.

Some patients who have a pheo present with sudden blood pressure spikes, while others present with ordinary hypertension or even low blood pressure. And in others, it is found purely coincidentally on an abdominal MRI or CT scan performed for reasons having nothing to do with hypertension.

Few doctors encounter a patient with this tumor in their entire career, and only one in one hundred patients with paroxysmal (episodic) hypertension turn out to have a pheo. If you have paroxysmal hypertension, your physician should do a screening blood or urine test for a pheo, although it is much more likely that you have "pseudopheochromocytoma," a form of neurogenic hypertension driven by psychological factors (chapter 11).

The most widely used screening tests consist of measurement of adrenaline and noradrenaline, or of their metabolites (metanephrines and normetanephrines) in blood or urine. Mildly elevated blood or urine levels are common, and usually are not indicative of a pheo. A very high level strongly suggests a pheo, and warrants an MRI to look for the tumor and a referral to a specialist for further management, which usually involves surgery to remove this potentially life-threatening tumor. The details of management of this rare tumor lie beyond the scope of this book.

13

HYPERTENSION IN
THE ELDERLY

Treating older patients with hypertension differs from treating younger patients. They respond a bit differently to the medications, the target blood pressure is different, and side effects can greatly affect the quality of life for the remaining years of their lives. Being on the right medication is extremely important.

Over two thirds of people over the age of sixty have hypertension, and one rule of thumb is that 77 percent of those above age seventy-seven have hypertension.[1] Most require medication to lower their blood pressure to a desired range.

I see many hypertensive patients who are in their seventies, eighties, and nineties, whose lives have been greatly affected by their medication. Side effects are just one issue. Another issue is confusion about what blood pressure level to aim for. A blood pressure that is normal, but too low for that individual, can cause weakness, tiredness, dizziness, and an increased risk of falling.

I encounter many older patients who feel tired and don't realize that their medication is the cause, assuming instead that it is just age and that there is nothing they can do about it. Some believe wrongly that tiredness is an unavoidable side effect of treatment.

Treating hypertension in patients above the age of eighty has been shown to prevent strokes and heart failure.[2] Does it prevent the progression of Alzheimer's disease? No, if Alzheimer's has already set in, it is too late. The cow is out of the barn. However, treating hypertension at a younger age reduces the likelihood of developing vascular dementia years later. Just one more reason to get your hypertension under control before the damage is done.

YOU MAY BE ON MORE MEDICATION THAN YOU NEED

Many elderly patients are on more medication than they need. In many who regard the blood pressure measurement as a gauge of risk of stroke, fear raises blood pressure in the moment that it is measured.

Also, as we get older, our arteries stiffen, and with stiffer arteries, our blood pressure fluctuates more. That is why, as we age, almost everyone has occasional high readings. If we treated everyone who had an occasional high reading, we would be, and are, treating too many people.

If your blood pressure was usually normal and your doctor started medication because one day it was high, you might not need the medication. If it was consistently normal on medication, but one day it was elevated and your doctor increased the medication, you probably didn't need the extra medication. Your doctor should obtain additional readings, or encourage you to obtain readings at home, before committing you to a permanent increase in medication.

Another reason for overmedication is that many doctors add medications without ever stopping those that didn't work. If you are taking several medications and your blood pressure is under control, ask your doctor if he can reduce or stop one or two of them. Worst case, your blood pressure may increase a bit, and you can resume the previous medication, knowing that you truly need it. It is rarely dangerous to do this, unless you have other underlying conditions that demand uninterrupted strict blood pressure control.

You also might be on a higher dose of your medication than you need. As we age, because of slower drug metabolism and excretion by our liver and kidneys, a given dose results in higher blood levels of many drugs. I generally try to start at a lower dose in older patients, and build it up if needed.

Few patients truly need four or five medications. If you are on that many, you might be on the wrong medications or on more medication than you truly need.

YOU MAY BE ON THE WRONG MEDICATION

Different people need different medication. You might be on a good drug, but it might not be the right one for you, leaving you with either persisting elevation of your blood pressure or side effects that you need not be living with, or both.

As I've discussed, there are clues that tell us which drug is right for you (chapter 9). If you need a diuretic and are not on one, your blood pressure might not come down even if your doctor prescribes four other medications. If you have neurogenic hypertension (chapter 9), your blood pressure might not normalize without an alpha- and beta-blocker, no matter how high a diuretic dose your doctor prescribes.

PICKING THE RIGHT BLOOD PRESSURE MEDICATIONS

When a younger patient is started on medication, most drug classes are equally effective in lowering blood pressure. On average, a diuretic, CCB, ACEI, or beta-blocker will lower blood pressure by the same amount. But in any given individual, they don't all lower blood pressure the same; one drug class will lower blood pressure much more than another. The trick is selecting the drug class most likely to work, as outlined in chapter 9.

In older patients the situation is different (table 13.1). We know that some drug classes work better than others. As we get older, sodium/volume is more commonly the main cause of hypertension, largely because with aging our kidneys are less efficient in excreting sodium. Consistent with this, in older patients, diuretics and CCBs have been shown to lower blood pressure more than ACEIs or ARBs.[3] Large trials have confirmed the effectiveness of CCBs and diuretics in reducing the risk of cardiovascular events.[4, 5]

That is why a diuretic or CCB should usually be the first choice. If the blood pressure doesn't come down to normal, then an ACEI or ARB can be added as the second drug. An exception though may lie in individuals with a truly low sodium intake, in whom an ACEI or ARB is more likely to work better, and is a reasonable alternative for initial treatment.

Again, these recommendations are not absolute. Some individuals respond better to an ACEI or ARB. We cannot predict reponse with certainty. But what we can do is improve the odds that we get it right with the first drug, and hopefully avoid the need for adding a second drug.

Table 13.1   Preferred drugs for treatment of hypertension in the elderly

Initial treatment: Diuretic or CCB
Add-on drug: ACEI, ARB, DRI, or beta-blocker

WHAT TARGET BLOOD PRESSURE
IS THE RIGHT TARGET?

This is an area of considerable controversy. In younger patients, the guide-lines call for an office systolic blood pressure below 140 (I usually aim for readings below 130) or a home systolic pressure below 130. Ideally, even 120 or less. But as we age, it is not clear that striving for the same low blood pressure is helpful in terms of longevity or quality of life. Piling on medica-tion after medication to achieve a systolic pressure of 130 rather than 140 in the patient over eighty might achieve no benefit, while increasing side effects.

Each of us is different, and, as we age, different people tolerate a differ-ent blood pressure. If an eighty-five-year-old feels well with a systolic pres-sure of 150, and weak and dizzy if it is lowered to 130, I would leave it at 150, especially since there is no proof yet that at that age, lowering systolic blood pressure to below 130 provides a better outcome.

We know from studies like the HYVET (Hypertension in the Very El-derly Trial) that in octogenarians with a systolic blood pressure above 160 mm, lowering it to under 160 is beneficial.[2] Many doctors don't realize though that we don't have evidence yet that lowering it further to below 140 provides more benefit than harm. If you are eighty-five and don't feel well at a systolic pressure of 125, you might need to be on less medication and at a higher blood pressure.

I suspect the answer also depends on the individual. A frail eighty-five-year-old might be harmed, while a vigorous eighty-five-year-old with a life expectancy of many years might benefit from a lower blood pressure level.

Then should your doctor aim to get your systolic pressure down to the 150s or down to the 130s? At the moment it's a judgment call. There is no clearly established right or wrong. I believe it is worthwhile trying to lower your blood pressure to below 140, as long as it can be done without side effects and without requiring a truckload of pills.

One final, but crucial, point: although doctors usually measure blood pressure in the seated position, measuring it in the standing position is also very important. If your standing blood pressure is low and you feel weak and dizzy, then you are on too much medication regardless of what your sitting blood pressure is. If your systolic blood pressure is 150 when you are sitting, but it falls to 110 and you feel dizzy when you stand up, your medication should be reduced, not increased. If you aren't feeling well on the medication, make sure to check your standing blood pressure, either at the doctor's office or at home.

AVOIDABLE SIDE EFFECTS

Too many elderly patients are on too many medications. And the more medication you are on, the more side effects you are likely to be experiencing (table 13.2). Also important, some medications are more likely than others to cause side effects, as discussed below.

In my experience, fatigue is a hugely important and common problem. As I have discussed in previous chapters, certain medications are notorious for causing fatigue—in particular, beta-blockers, clonidine, and the nondihydropyridine CCBs diltiazem (Cardizem) and verapamil (Isoptin, Calan) (table 13.3). Whether it is tiredness, a lack of pep, or the sense that you have to push yourself anytime you want to do something, it can be due to your medication. Even if you think you feel well, you might not realize how much you have been slowed down. Don't assume it is your age.

If you are on a beta-blocker and feel a lack of pep, ask your doctor if you truly need to be taking a beta-blocker. **Millions of people who are taking a beta-blocker for their hypertension don't really need to be on one.** But don't stop it on your own. This should be done gradually and under the supervision of a physician.

Likewise, many elderly patients taking diltiazem (Cardizem) or verapamil (Isoptin, Calan) for their hypertension don't need those particular drugs. If you are experiencing fatigue, your doctor can easily switch to another drug class, or to a dihydropyridine CCB, such as amlodipine (Norvasc) or

Table 13.2 Common avoidable side effects

Tiredness
Lack of energy
Mental dullness
Dizziness
Constipation
Swelling in the legs
Hyponatremia (low blood sodium level)

Table 13.3 Antihypertensive drugs most likely to cause fatigue

- Beta-blockers
- Nondihydropyridine CCBs (e.g., diltiazem [Cardizem], verapamil [Isoptin, Calan])
- Central alpha-agonists (e.g., clonidine [Catapres])

nifedipine (Procardia), that don't cause tiredness. And drugs such as clonidine (Catapres) cause fatigue (and dry mouth) in most people and are one
of the *last* drugs I would choose for an elderly patient or for anyone. **Very
few patients who are on clonidine need to be on it!**

Most individuals in their upper seventies and eighties complain of some
degree of memory loss. I don't think blood pressure medication commonly
worsens it, but occasionally it does. Mental dullness, a slowness of thinking,
is another possible side effect. Drugs that get into the brain can cause these.
In my experience, beta-blockers that get into the brain, such as labetalol
(Trandate, Normodyne), propranolol (Inderal), metoprolol (Toprol), and
carvedilol (Coreg) (chapter 6), can do this, particularly in individuals who
metabolize beta-blockers very slowly (chapter 6). If you are on such a drug
and your thinking or memory seems slower, the only way you can find out if
the drug is the cause is if your doctor is willing to do the experiment of stopping the drug, reducing the dose, or switching to a different drug (chapter
6). It is worth finding out.

The CCBs, particularly in older patients, are frequent causes of constipation and fluid retention in the legs (edema). Sadly, **most patients suffering constipation from a nondihydropyridine CCB (diltiazem or
verapamil) don't need to be on a CCB!** Aggravation of constipation is
the last thing an older patient needs.

Fluid retention in the legs (edema) can bother patients in a number of
ways. It can cause itching, redness, and rash in the skin (stasis dermatitis).
It can make your legs feel heavier. More important, when you go to bed
at night, the more fluid you have in your legs, the more will reenter your
bloodstream once you are off your feet and the more frequently you will
need to urinate in the middle of the night. The interruption of sleep is not
a trivial problem.

If edema is bothersome, switching from a CCB to a diuretic will usually
reduce the edema while controlling the hypertension. When I see a new
patient who needs to start medication but has some edema, a diuretic is
usually a better choice, as it will reduce rather than increase edema.

As I discussed in chapter 3, the diuretics can lower not only the potassium
level but also the blood sodium level. This serious and common problem
affects almost exclusively patients over the age of seventy, particularly those
with a copious water intake. A low sodium concentration (hyponatremia)
can cause weakness, nausea, and confusion, and, if extremely low, vomiting
and even coma and neurological damage.

The cause is not a lack of sodium but an excess of water. You are at high
risk of developing hyponatremia if you are older than seventy, have a *high*

water intake (aging kidneys are less able to excrete excess water), and *are taking a thiazide or potassium-sparing diuretic*, which causes excretion of relatively more sodium than water. Although a low salt diet is healthy, when it is combined with a high water intake and a thiazide diuretic, it can contribute to hyponatremia. The treatment of this condition, and guidance as to which diuretics are least likely to cause hyponatremia, is discussed in chapter 3.

The important point is that the dictum that you need to drink eight glasses of water a day is wrong, and can be dangerous if you are over seventy and especially if you are taking a thiazide diuretic. Some people— for example, those with a history of kidney stones or recurrent urinary infections—do need a higher fluid intake. And obviously, heavy sweating requires fluid replacement. But otherwise excessive water intake can do more harm than good.

When patients ask how much fluid they should take in, the answer is actually very simple. In most cases, our body knows when we need fluid. All you have to do is listen to your body. You don't have to drink more fluid because you "think" it is the right thing to do. In most people two quarts a day, or even less, is more than ample.

To summarize, many elderly patients are on too many medications, on too high a dosage, or on the wrong medications. Adverse effects that reduce quality of life are easily avoidable by choosing medications that don't cause them. The goal is to control the blood pressure with the fewest number of medications by picking the drugs most likely to work and least likely to cause side effects. And if your blood pressure is normal, your doctor should make the attempt to reduce your medication.

14

ALCOHOL, COFFEE, AND COMMONLY USED OVER-THE-COUNTER DRUGS

If you have hypertension, many doctors rigidly forbid the use of medications that can increase blood pressure. But is it really necessary to rigidly forbid the use of drugs that many of us really need and benefit from, such as decongestants, anti-inflammatory drugs, and others? In this chapter, I will review the effects on blood pressure of commonly used agents, such as coffee, alcohol, cigarettes, anti-inflammatory drugs, cold remedies, and birth control pills. Can people who have hypertension use these drugs? Are they safe or not?

DECONGESTANTS

What I hate most about having a cold is the nasal congestion. I can't breathe freely. And I know that after a few days, my congested sinuses might start to ache, and I might end up needing an antibiotic if they end up infected due to lack of drainage. Fortunately, there are effective decongestants and anti-inflammatory sprays that can prevent those problems. And decongestant sprays, such as oxymetazoline (Afrin), can relieve the congestion within minutes.

My experience tells me that sinus congestion is not treated adequately in many hypertensive patients. Many doctors tell their hypertensive patients that they cannot use a decongestant spray, because decongestants can raise blood pressure. I see patients who have suffered needlessly and then ended up with sinus infections that required antibiotics. Or they were given an antibiotic right away, which often was unnecessary and of no help. The timely use of a decongestant, particularly when a steroid or antihistamine spray is also given, can allow drainage, relieve symptoms, and prevent development of the bacterial sinus infections that do require antibiotics.

Banning decongestants in hypertensive patients is usually unnecessary because in people with ordinary hypertension that is under control, they are rarely dangerous. The risk is not zero, but it is extremely low. I am comfortable prescribing them in most of my hypertensive patients. Although many doctors worry that the decongestants can cause a major spike in blood pressure, such spikes are very uncommon.[1] Any elevation that does occur is usually mild and usually too trivial to justify withholding helpful treatment. Also, if you are taking blood pressure medication and your blood pressure is normal or near normal, an increase in blood pressure of maybe a few millimeters for just a few days is truly a trivial matter. For extra safety, you can monitor your blood pressure at home and stop the drug if your blood pressure increases to a significant degree.

If your blood pressure is only slightly elevated, I would still prescribe a decongestant, but would recommend monitoring your blood pressure at home. If your blood pressure is significantly elevated, it is probably safer to avoid the decongestants; but you shouldn't be in that situation, as your blood pressure should be under control.

Although decongestants can usually be safely used if your blood pressure is under control, caution is necessary if you have some other condition that could be affected by a decongestant, such as angina, abnormal heart rhythm, aneurysm, or others. That is why I recommend that before you take a decongestant, you first ask your physician if it is okay.

The most widely used decongestants are sprays like oxymetazoline (Afrin), or pills like pseudoephedrine (Sudafed). I like prescribing Afrin because it relieves congestion immediately and is available over-the-counter. But it should be used for only a couple of days, and I recommend to patients a maximum of two days at a time, because longer use can result in rebound congestion when you try to stop it.

There are also sprays that shrink membranes and relieve congestion that don't raise blood pressure at all. These include steroid sprays, such as fluticasone (Flonase), mometasone (Nasonex), and budesonide (Rhinocort), and antihistamine sprays, such as azelastine (Astelin). The steroid sprays though take a couple of days before their effect kicks in.

When my hypertensive patients ask for treatment for nasal congestion from a cold or from allergies, my favorite recommendation is a combination of two sprays: a steroid spray to be taken for a week, with the expectation that it will take two or three days before its effect kicks in, along with a decongestant spray, such as oxymetazoline (Afrin), to be taken only for the first two days to provide immediate relief until the steroid spray kicks in. When patients come to me with nasal congestion and ask for an antibiotic, I usually recommend the two sprays instead, with the proviso that if they don't improve or if they develop fever, I'll prescribe the antibiotic. Very few end up calling.

NONSTEROIDAL ANTI-INFLAMMATORY DRUGS (NSAIDS)

The NSAIDs are widely used for pain or fever. Millions of people with arthritis depend on them, and I have many patients who could barely function without them.

The studies show that NSAIDs raise blood pressure, on average by a couple of millimeters.[2, 3] In some people they don't affect the blood pressure, but in others, they can raise it by 10 millimeters or more. If you have hypertension, is it okay to take an NSAID? Many doctors won't prescribe one.

My answer is a qualified yes. If you have arthritis or chronic pain from other causes and can manage with other drugs, such as acetaminophen (Tylenol), I wouldn't prescribe an NSAID. But if you cannot manage without an NSAID, I would prescribe one and tweak the blood pressure medication if necessary. And of course, I would recommend using the NSAID for as brief a time as possible. Use it on bad days or bad weeks, and skip it or use acetaminophen (Tylenol) when the pain is not so bad.

I ask hypertensive patients who are taking an NSAID to monitor their blood pressure at home. In most patients, it changes very little; an increase in systolic pressure from 123 to 126 is barely noticeable. As with the decongestants, I am more wary about using NSAIDs in patients whose blood pressure is not under control, but in most of my patients, the blood pressure is under control. Also, studies suggest that the COX-2 inhibitor celecoxib (Celebrex) is less likely to raise blood pressure than are the NSAIDs, with an equivalent pain-reducing effect.

If you take an NSAID and your blood pressure increases significantly, what should your doctor do? Stop the NSAID if possible. But if you truly need it, I would continue taking it and would adjust the blood pressure medication.

The drugs most likely to help overcome NSAID-induced blood pressure elevation are the diuretics and the CCBs. When you take an NSAID, your kidneys hold on to sodium and fluid, which is why most people gain a few pounds while taking them. Increasing your diuretic helps negate the fluid retention. The alternative is a CCB, which relaxes arteries and lowers blood pressure, but might add to the fluid retention.

NSAIDs can increase blood potassium level, lower sodium level, or reduce kidney function. These should be checked by your physician, particularly if you are older, have reduced kidney function, or are taking a diuretic, ACE, or ARB. **If you have abnormal kidney function, you should usually avoid use of NSAIDs.** You should take an NSAID only under the close supervision of a doctor (even naproxen [Aleve] and ibuprofen [Advil] can cause problems) and make sure to have blood tests to check your kidney function, sodium, and potassium within a few days of starting it.

Finally, in recent years, highly publicized studies have indicated that use of NSAIDs is associated with an increased risk of cardiovascular events.[4] The studies have not identified any particular NSAID as clearly safer than the others. This also argues for minimizing use of NSAIDs and limiting their use to shorter periods when you truly need them, rather than taking them daily for years. That said, if you have severe or disabling pain and NSAIDs do the best job of relieving the pain for you, then an NSAID is worth the small increase in cardiovascular risk. But I would try to minimize the cardiovascular risk by monitoring and controlling your blood pressure, as well as other cardiovascular risk factors, such as cholesterol level, smoking, obesity, etc.

ALCOHOL

Here's a common misconception: having an alcoholic drink raises your blood pressure. It doesn't. **A drink or two actually lowers your blood pressure!** Alcohol is a vasodilator—it relaxes arteries and lowers blood pressure. Not to mention its relaxing effect on the mind.

When a patient with well-controlled hypertension calls me because he is worried about an elevated reading, in which case it is usually unnecessary and unwise to increase the blood pressure medication, I sometimes even suggest having a drink. The blood pressure usually quickly falls! The effect is sometimes sizeable, with systolic blood pressure falling 30 mm or more.

Why do so many people think alcohol raises blood pressure? Probably because in excessive amounts it does. It raises blood pressure by stimulating the sympathetic nervous system (SNS) (chapter 2). Also people who become dependent on alcohol frequently experience alcohol withdrawal, which also stimulates the SNS and raises blood pressure.

When alcohol abuse is responsible for resistant hypertension, the most appropriate solution is to reduce or stop drinking. If a patient cannot stop drinking, I prescribe blood pressure drugs that block the effects of the SNS, specifically an alpha/beta-blocker combination (chapter 9).

Ironically, my concern about alcohol is usually about a fall in blood pressure, rather than an increase. It can *lower* your blood pressure too much. If you are taking vasodilating drugs, particularly an alpha-blocker, the added vasodilating effect of alcohol can lower your blood pressure even further, causing weakness, dizziness, and even fainting. If you are on blood pressure medication and have a drink and then feel dizzy, sit down. It'll pass. Would I recommend you never drink? No, but be careful.

BIRTH CONTROL PILLS

Birth control pills, which contain a combination of estrogen and progesterone, can elevate blood pressure, sometimes severely, even in women with no history of hypertension, through stimulation of the renin-angiotensin system (chapter 2). For reasons we don't understand, the hypertension can first develop even after months or years of taking the pill. Women with a history of hypertension are at greater risk of developing hypertension, including severe hypertension. It was hoped that pills with a lower amount of estrogen would not raise blood pressure, but it turned out that they can.

If you are taking the pill and your blood pressure has risen to the hypertensive range, you should usually stop it. If your blood pressure falls back to normal, it is clear that the pill was the cause. Many doctors don't realize though that it can take up to six months for the blood pressure elevation to resolve. Two months may be too short an interval to decide whether stopping the pill will make a difference.

If you truly need the pill despite the blood pressure increase, for example, to prevent severe pain caused by endometriosis (growth of uterine tissue outside the uterus), treatment with an ACEI or ARB to antagonize the effect of the pill on the RAS is usually effective. If the blood pressure is controlled with the medication, I reluctantly go along with the patient's wish to continue taking the pill. If not, it should be stopped. I also insist that the patient monitor her blood pressure at home at least once a week.

What about estrogen-replacement therapy during menopause? If anything, estrogen replacement lowers blood pressure, although some studies indicate it may increase the risk of stroke due to effects on the clotting system.

CIGARETTES

This section is plain and simple. Cigarettes raise blood pressure in almost everyone, usually about 5 to 10 mm or more for about a half hour.[5] This happens with every cigarette you smoke. Worse, the vasoconstriction caused by nicotine, combined with hypertension, is a wicked combination and profoundly accelerates development of arteriosclerosis that leads to heart attacks and strokes. If you have hypertension, smoking is about the worst thing you can do.

CAFFEINE

Caffeine is a more interesting issue. Many patients ask me about coffee, and the answer was quite murky until recently.

Does coffee drinking raise your blood pressure? Conventional wisdom used to be that the occasional cup could raise your blood pressure, but habitual drinkers seemed to adjust to it, with little effect on blood pressure. It turns out that that was wrong.

A recent and interesting study provided the answer[6]: the effect of coffee on your blood pressure depends on how you metabolize caffeine, which is genetically determined. If you are a rapid metabolizer, the caffeine is gone quickly and there will be no effect on your blood pressure. If you are a slow metabolizer, you will sustain high blood levels of caffeine, which stimulates the sympathetic nervous system and elevates blood pressure, 5 to 10 mm or more, cup after cup.

How can you tell whether caffeine will affect your blood pressure? There is no blood test. The only way is to do the experiment at home with your blood pressure monitor. Check your blood pressure after sitting for five minutes, drink one or two cups of coffee, and then recheck it in an hour or two. You might want to repeat the experiment a couple of times to be sure.

Is decaf okay? Yes. Tea? Tea and cola each has caffeine but less than half of what coffee contains. Chocolate also has caffeine, but much less; it is negligible unless you binge on chocolate (table 14.1).

Table 14.1   Milligrams of caffeine in caffeine-containing drinks

Coffee	103	Tea	40
Instant coffee	57	Instant tea	30
Decaf coffee	2	Decaf tea	1
Cola	31–70	Chocolate bar	10

SEX AND EXERCISE

Patients frequently ask me about the effects of blood pressure medications on exercise and on sex. In the first half of this chapter, I will deal with the relationship between blood pressure medication and sex. Does medication interfere with desire and with sexual function? Are some medications worse offenders than others? Is sex dangerous with uncontrolled hypertension? Are drugs like sildenafil (Viagra) safe? In the second half of this chapter, I will discuss exercise: Does the medication affect exercise capacity? Is one medication worse than another? Is exercise dangerous? What is the best exercise? What about weightlifting?

ANTIHYPERTENSIVE MEDICATION AND SEX

Does antihypertensive medication interfere with sexual function and desire? Does it cause erectile dysfunction (ED)? The answer is yes, but it's not that simple.

Antihypertensive Medication and Erectile Dysfunction (ED)

As we age, we all develop some degree of narrowing of small arteries throughout our body. Narrowing and dysfunction of the small arteries that supply our sexual organs leads to ED. With age, a majority of people eventually develop ED.

Anything that accelerates the aging of our arteries, such as hypertension, smoking, diabetes, hypercholesterolemia, and obesity, will lower the age at which ED occurs. If you have longstanding untreated hypertension, particularly if you have been a smoker or have any of the other conditions, you are likely to have narrowing and dysfunction of your small arteries; and if you don't already have ED, you are on your way to it.

The treatment of hypertension affects this circulation in two ways. The first is good; the second, not so good. The good news: lowering your blood pressure with medication helps protect your small arteries. The bad news: if your small arteries are already narrowed, reducing blood pressure with medication can reduce the flow of blood through them, reducing erectile function. This can happen no matter what antihypertensive medicine you are taking.

Most, but not all, patients with intact erectile function are unaffected by blood pressure lowering; those with small artery damage are more likely to be affected. If a blood pressure drug causes ED, stopping it can improve sexual function, but the higher blood pressure levels will lead to further damage to your small arteries, and ultimately to ED, as well as to a greater risk of cardiovascular events. In other words, you are caught between a rock and a soft place! So in this situation, treating your hypertension may involve a trade-off: it will reduce your risk of stroke and heart attack and can add years to your life, but it might reduce your erectile function. Fortunately, we have the option of taking pills that address ED, and they do work.

Do Some Medications Cause ED More Than Others?   Are some drug classes more likely to cause ED than others? Yes, particularly those that reduce blood flow, such as beta-blockers; those with hormonal effects, such as spironolactone; and those with effects in the brain, such as clonidine (Catapres) (table 15.1).

The diuretics reduce blood volume a bit but are less likely to cause ED than they were decades ago when they were used at very high doses. Beta-blockers reduce the amount of blood pumped by the heart and also constrict the small arteries, reducing blood flow. A new beta-blocker, nebivolol (Bystolic), dilates the small arteries and might be less likely to cause ED.

Table 15.1   Blood pressure medications most likely to cause ED

- Beta-blockers
- Central alpha-agonists (e.g., clonidine)
- Spironolactone
- Diuretics

Drugs like clonidine have very prominent effects in the central nervous system and often interfere with sexual function.

The potassium-sparing diuretic spironolactone (Aldactone) (chapter 3), which binds to aldosterone receptors and blocks the effects of that hormone, also binds to sex hormone receptors, and can cause ED independently of its effect on blood pressure. If this occurs, there are two potassium-sparing diuretics that can be used in its place, eplerenone (Inspra) and amiloride (Midamor). Eplerenone (Inspra), which also blocks the effect of aldosterone, is less likely to bind sex hormone receptors and to cause ED. Amiloride (Midamor) doesn't bind any hormone receptors.

Which antihypertensive drugs are least likely to cause ED? Those which dilate arteries: ACEIs, ARBs, and CCBs. The ACEIs can reduce testosterone levels resulting in ED, but this is very uncommon.

If you are taking a diuretic and are experiencing ED, your doctor can replace it with a CCB, or reduce the dose if your blood pressure is well controlled. If you are taking a beta-blocker, in many cases he can safely replace it with an ACEI or ARB. Of course, if you truly require a diuretic or beta-blocker, it should not be stopped.

The best advice: if you have hypertension and normal sexual function and want to reduce your chances of developing ED, get your blood pressure under control, stop smoking, lose weight, exercise, and, if you have diabetes or hypercholesterolemia, get them under control. And treat hypertension early, before it causes the small artery damage that causes ED.

Sexual Desire

I am limited in what I can say about libido and blood pressure medication because there is much less in the medical literature about libido than about erectile function. It is harder to measure. Also, it seems as if hypertension researchers have only recently discovered that women have a libido.

I would suspect that drugs that have effects in the brain, such as the central alpha-agonists, like clonidine, are more likely to affect libido than other drugs. Beta-blockers might also affect libido. But again, there is little available in the literature.

Is Sex Dangerous If Your Blood Pressure Is Elevated?

Sexual intercourse increases your heart rate and blood pressure substantially. In most people, this is not a problem—our blood pressure routinely spikes during many activities, such as running, lifting a heavy box, or getting angry. However, if you have uncontrolled hypertension, with a higher baseline blood pressure to start with, the peak blood pressure will also be higher.

Fortunately, even when our blood pressure spikes, it is extremely unlikely to cause serious problems, such as bursting a blood vessel in the brain. However, if you have problems such as coronary artery disease, there is an increased risk of developing chest pain (angina) due to the heart's increased need for oxygen while the heart rate and blood pressure are increased. Rarely a heart attack can occur, due to a slightly increased risk of rupturing a plaque in your coronary artery.

The bottom line: if your blood pressure is very high, should you engage in sex? You are taking a risk, albeit a small one. Should you see your doctor? Yes. Not because sex is dangerous but because your blood pressure needs attention.

Viagra, Cialis, and Levitra

In most people with hypertension and ED, they work. Are they safe if your blood pressure is somewhat elevated? Yes, they don't raise blood pressure; they actually lower it. Several of my patients tell me their best blood pressure readings occur after taking Viagra.

Is it safe to take them if you are taking blood pressure medication? Yes, except if you are taking nitroglycerin, because of the risk of excessive vasodilation and fall in blood pressure. There had been concern about their use in patients who were taking an alpha-blocker (e.g., doxazosin [Cardura] or terazosin [Hytrin]), although it is currently considered safe to use them. Even so, if dizziness develops, I would recommend checking the blood pressure and holding off further use until consulting with your physician.

One recommendation: if you are on any blood pressure medication, or even if you are not, the first time you try any of these drugs, start with the lowest-dose pill. It is always the safest way. Or take half of the higher-dose pill, and if it works, you've got a twofer.

ANTIHYPERTENSIVE MEDICATION AND EXERCISE

Some questions come up again and again. Is exercise safe if you have hypertension? What is the best exercise? Is weight lifting okay or not? What medications are least likely to interfere with athletic performance or endurance?

What Does Your Blood Pressure Do During Exercise?

With aerobic exercise, such as running, it is normal for blood pressure to increase to about 180 or 190/70 to 90. The increase is mainly in systolic pressure. If you have hypertension, your blood pressure will start out higher and end up higher. If your hypertension is treated, your peak blood pressure will also be lowered.

During isometric exercise, like weight lifting, both systolic and diastolic blood pressure increase considerably while bearing down and can reach as high as 230/120 even if you've never had hypertension! But even this high level rarely puts you in danger. These elevations are brief and are part of normal blood pressure fluctuation. I wouldn't say it is good for you, but normally you are not in danger. Even Olympic weight lifters don't suffer strokes while weight lifting.

Do these elevations, if they occur again and again over years, harm you over the long run? We really don't know for sure, but I've not seen evidence that they do.

Can You Exercise If You Have Hypertension?

Exercise is good for everyone, and if you have hypertension, it is even more important. **Every study shows that over time aerobic exercise lowers blood pressure and, better yet, reduces the risk of cardiovascular events by about half.**

If you have hypertension and your blood pressure is under control or is only mildly elevated, any exercise is safe. If it is quite high, say 160/100 or higher, it is probably better to avoid strenuous exercise until it is in a better range.

What About Weight Lifting?

Most doctors routinely warn hypertensive patients not to lift weights. Is this restriction necessary?

Weight lifting would not be my first choice, because of the brief blood pressure surges, but I have to admit that there is no clear evidence of negative consequence. And weight lifting is important for maintaining muscle tone.

Every study shows that regular aerobic exercise lowers blood pressure readings over time. Surprisingly, studies also show that regular weight lifting, even though it raises blood pressure in the moment, also lowers blood pressure a bit over time.[1]

Then if you have hypertension, is weight lifting okay? The answer is yes, although I don't think serious bodybuilding is a good idea. As with everything else, moderation is best.

Which Is the Best Exercise?

Many patients ask me whether I think running, swimming, power walking, or biking is the best exercise, or is it something else? My answer is simple: what is most important is that you exercise on a regular basis. The best exercise is one that you enjoy; if you enjoy it, you are more likely to keep doing it.

My exercise is running, and I have been running for over thirty years. However, for many patients I think running is the wrong exercise. If you are very overweight, the wear and tear and strain of running is a problem, and you will be at risk of injury, particularly if you are a little older and are not used to regular exercise. Power walking, biking, or swimming may be kinder to your body.

Which Medication Is Least Likely to Interfere with Exercise Endurance?

This is a question that I face most often with young patients, particularly competitive athletes. Their very real concern is that medication can reduce their stamina.

The effect of beta-blockers on exercise capacity is complex. They reduce our ability to increase heart rate and cardiac output. Beta-blockers also constrict arteries, which can reduce the amount of blood and oxygen delivered to exercising muscle. In general I try to avoid beta-blockers in athletes.

Another problem is that beta-blockers reduce one's desire to do physical exercise—you can do the exercise, but you just don't feel like it. The same exercise requires more effort when you are taking a beta-blocker. And reduced exercise reduces fitness.

The ACEIs, ARBs, CCBs, and diuretics are less likely than beta-blockers to interfere with exercise capacity. However, I am concerned that a diuretic, in combination with the copious sweating of endurance sports, can cause dehydration. In long-distance runners, for example, I might avoid the diuretics or prescribe the lowest possible dose, and/or have the patient skip the diuretic on days of hard or long workouts or competition.

Extreme Endurance Sports

Extreme endurance sports, such as marathons and triathlons, pose risks even to the healthiest competitors. They obviously pose at least as much risk in hypertensive patients. They carry a risk of dehydration, low blood pressure, heat stroke, and other complications. Well-controlled hypertension probably adds little risk. But the more severe the history of hypertension, and the more medication required to control it, the more likely it is that the risk is increased.

Are extreme endurance sports safe in the hypertensive patient who is on medication and has a normal blood pressure? My answer would be the following: I believe strongly that exercise is important and healthful. But I believe equally strongly that extreme endurance sports are not more beneficial than a regular exercise regimen, and cause tremendous wear and tear damage. I wouldn't recommend extreme endurance sports for patients who don't have hypertension, and I certainly don't recommend them for patients who do, whether they are taking medication or not.

16

REDUCING MEDICATIONS AND CUTTING MEDICATION COSTS

If you have uncomplicated hypertension that is under control, and you think you are on too many medications, you are not alone. Millions of people are on more medications than they need, with one or more of their medications not doing anything for them. They absolutely could reduce their drugs and drug costs without any harmful impact on their hypertension. In this chapter, I will review how.

"ONCE ON MEDICATION ALWAYS ON MEDICATION"— TRUE OR FALSE?

I see many patients who are under the impression that once they start medication, they must stay on medication forever and can never stop it. This is partly, but not entirely, true. Medication doesn't cure hypertension; it controls it. If you stop medication that is working and that you need, your blood pressure will usually increase, whether within days, weeks, or months. That is why if medications are doing the job, we usually continue them. That said, it is often possible to reduce or stop medications that you don't truly need (table 16.1).

Table 16.1   Questions regarding the safety of reducing medication

1. How severe was your hypertension before it was treated?
2. Do you have other medical conditions that argue for stringent blood pressure control?

IS IT SAFE TO REDUCE YOUR MEDICATION?

Many patients are concerned that their blood pressure might spike if they reduce or stop their medication. The good news is that that is unlikely to happen when medication is stopped in an appropriate way, under the supervision of a physician, and, optimally, if you monitor your blood pressure at home. The worst case: your blood pressure will go up a bit, and you would restart the medication.

If your blood pressure is well controlled, it is usually safe to try to reduce dosage and eliminate unnecessary medications. However, in certain circumstances, I would be cautious about reducing medications. If you previously had very severe hypertension, there is a greater chance of severe blood pressure elevation if you reduce medication. Fortunately though, with good blood pressure control, over time even severe hypertension becomes easier to control and requires less medication, allowing for reduction in medication. Your physician should go slow though, and you should follow your home blood pressure carefully, at least every other day if not every day initially.

Another reason for caution would be if you have a condition such as angina, heart failure, or severely reduced kidney function, conditions that could worsen with loss of blood pressure control. Even if you are doing well, it might be best to leave well enough alone and not reduce the medication. If you have diabetes or kidney disease, we aim for the best blood pressure possible to prevent worsening of kidney function. Unless you are having side effects, or your blood pressure is too low, it may be best to err on the side of too much rather than too little medication.

REASONS FOR OVERTREATMENT

There are two main reasons why you might not need some of the medication you are on: (1) you never really needed it and (2) you have made substantial lifestyle changes (table 16.2).

Table 16.2   Reasons why you might not need medication or might need less medication

---

A. **You never really needed all the medication you are on.**
- Anxiety about your blood pressure may be responsible for elevated readings in the doctor's office and/or at home.
- Your blood pressure has been measured incorrectly at the doctor's office and/ or at home.
- Your blood pressure elevation might have been temporary.
- Some of your medications are doing nothing and can be stopped.
- A stronger diuretic regimen can eliminate the need for some of your other medications.

B. **You have made substantial changes in your health habits.**
- You have changed your diet and/or exercise habits.
- You have lost weight.

You Never Really Needed as Much Medication as You Are Taking

In chapter 1, I discussed two circumstances that often lead to unnecessary treatment: white coat hypertension, and incorrect measurement of blood pressure, either in the doctor's office or at home. Your blood pressure might be lower than you or your doctor think, and you might not need all the medication you are on.

Temporary hypertension is another possibility. I have seen many patients whose blood pressure was elevated for days or weeks; then, without any treatment, it drifted down to normal and stayed normal. That is why it is not the standard recommendation to initiate or increase medication based on mild elevation on a single occasion. Unfortunately, some doctors are quick to treat; and when the blood pressure returns to normal, the improvement is wrongly attributed to the medication, which is then continued indefinitely.

What caused the temporary elevation? Perhaps a major stress, or a higher sodium intake than usual. Perhaps the blood pressure was checked at an extremely stressful moment, with elevation limited to that moment. Sometimes there is no obvious reason. Regardless, if your blood pressure had always been normal, mild elevation for several days does not automatically require initiation of, or an increase in, medication.

Many patients with well-controlled hypertension occasionally have an elevated reading. It is unnecessary to increase medication unless the blood pressure is extremely high or remains elevated either at home or at more than one visit. If your blood pressure, on medication, has been consistently normal, chances are nine out of ten that the readings will return to normal without any intervention.

Even if you truly need medication, you may be on more medications than you need. The most frequent cause: some of your medications are wrong for you and are doing nothing for your blood pressure. It is often worthwhile to try to eliminate medications that didn't help, if your blood pressure is now well controlled. If you have volume-mediated hypertension (chapters 2 and 9) and are on less of a diuretic than you need, the other drugs you are on might be doing little and might not be necessary. If you are on three or four drugs but not a diuretic, ask your doctor about starting a diuretic and about reducing other medications.

You Have Made Substantial Lifestyle Changes

If you have made serious changes in your eating and exercise habits, if you have reduced your salt intake and/or lost weight, there is a good chance that you will require less medication or even no medication. Ironically, the worse your diet was to start with or the more overweight you were, the greater the likelihood that you can reduce the amount of medication you need. If you were 40 pounds overweight, you can lower your blood pressure more than if you had only been 10 pounds overweight.

Making the necessary changes does not guarantee that you will be able to reduce or get off your medication, but it does increase the odds. Even if you can't, you have improved your health anyway. So you win, even if you have to remain on medication.

STOPPING MEDICATION SAFELY

When it comes to actually stopping medication, there is a right and wrong way (table 16.3).

Table 16.3   How to stop medication

1. Don't reduce your medication on your own.
2. Monitor your blood pressure regularly at home.
3. Reduce the dose gradually; taper medications that require tapering.
4. Don't overreact to a single elevated reading.
5. Beware: your blood pressure might remain normal for months and then rise.
6. Be vigilant in maintaining a healthy diet.

How to Stop Medication

Some dos and don'ts:

Don't reduce the medication on your own. If your physician feels you should not reduce or stop it, and you feel she is wrong, ask her to explain why you shouldn't.

Do monitor your blood pressure at home. During the first few weeks after reducing or stopping medication, I usually ask patients to monitor their blood pressure at home at least twice a week and, if the systolic blood pressure readings are averaging more than 10 millimeters or so higher, to either let me know or simply resume the previous medication or dose. Can medication be reduced without home monitoring? Yes, particularly if you have mild hypertension. But if you aren't monitoring your blood pressure at home, you will need more frequent visits to the doctor.

Stop one medication at a time, unless your blood pressure is on the low side. If your blood pressure increases after you have reduced or stopped a drug, resume it and try reducing a different one until you identify which drugs you need and which you don't.

In the case of certain medications, taper rather than abruptly stop them. Stopping certain medications suddenly can sometimes cause problems. Suddenly stopping medications such as clonidine can lead to a withdrawal syndrome with a rapid heart rate and severe elevation of blood pressure. Stopping a beta-blocker suddenly can cause agitation, a rapid heart rate, and even an abnormal heart rhythm. Under the supervision of your doctor, they should be tapered gradually to a minimum dose, with at least a few days at each step, before stopping them. Stopping a diuretic suddenly can cause fluid retention with a weight gain of several pounds. It is always best to reduce and stop a diuretic gradually (chapter 3).

Don't overreact to a single elevated reading. Everyone's blood pressure varies from day to day and from reading to reading. Seeing an elevated reading after you reduce or stop a medication does not mean that you need to go back to the original dose. It does mean that you need to continue monitoring your blood pressure to see whether or not it remains persistently higher.

A word of caution: many doctors and patients think that when you reduce or stop medication, if your blood pressure is destined to increase, it will do so within days, as soon as the drug is out of your system. Often that is not true. Your blood pressure can remain normal for weeks or months and then increase. Why? Because your medication, by normalizing your blood pressure, stopped the hypertensive process and even turned the clock back in terms of effects on the structure of your arteries. When you stop an effective drug, the hypertensive process starts over again, and the blood pressure can start to rise again months later. If you stop medication, you must continue to monitor your blood pressure. And, of course, if your need for medication was reduced because of changes in diet and exercise, your blood pressure can rise if you waver in these efforts.

HOW TO CUT DRUG COSTS

The drugs you take for your hypertension can cost thousands of dollars a year. If your health care plan is paying most of the costs, you are in good shape. If not, you might be paying a bundle. Whether it is your health care plan, or you, that is trying to cut costs, there are many ways to do so without compromising your care.

It is hard to convey the cost of the drugs, because every plan offers different prices. Tables 16.4, 16.5, and 16.6 present prices for a ninety-day supply of a sampling of medications. Table 16.4 compares prices for generic versus brand name and prices for drugs available online on drugstore.com and in Walmart plans. Table 16.5 lists prices for a sampling of combination drugs. Table 16.6 lists the drugs available at the discounted price program at Walmart with prices of $4 for a thirty-day supply and $10 for a ninety-day supply.

It is very difficult to list the prices because every drug plan has its own unique list of preferred drugs, their own set of prices, and their own policies regarding co-payments. In addition, prices are always changing. In view of that, I want to caution that some of the prices listed in the tables might be outdated by the time the book is published, might differ from prices listed elsewhere, or might just be wrong. The main message of the tables is not specific prices, but a few general principles: generic is much less costly than brand name. Brand name combination pills (pills that contain two or more drugs) will not save you money. Generic combination pills cost roughly the same as the drugs priced separately, but provide the convenience of one pill instead of two.

In addition, the manufacturers of some of the newer drugs offer rebate plans or reduced co-pay plans. Some also offer arrangements for reduced cost in case of hardship. These are worth inquiring about at your physician's office.

Nowadays, when we speak of cutting drug costs, the word Canada keeps coming up. There is no doubt that prices of drugs from Canada are lower. The drug might or might not reliably contain what it is supposed to contain, and, unfortunately, there is no way to be certain.

Table 16.4   Sampling of prices for a ninety-day supply of antihypertensive drugs

Drug class	Dose	Cost ($): Generic			Cost ($): Brand name	
Diuretics		Retail	Drugstore .com	Walmart	Retail	Drugstore .com
hydrochlorothia-zide (HCTZ)	25 mg		13	10		
chlorthalidone (Hygroton)	25 mg		46	10		
spironolactone (Aldactone)	25 mg	43	30	10	107	102
eplerenone (Inspra)	50 mg	384	276		493	425
furosemide (Lasix)	40 mg		18			58
torsemide (Demadex)	10 mg	66	60		118	110
Calcium channel blockers (CCBs)						
nifedipine (Procardia XL)	30 mg	124	114		237	211
amlodipine (Norvasc)	10 mg	222	24		338	300
diltiazem (Cardizem CD)	240 mg	192	121		616	557
Angiotensin-converting enzyme inhibitors (ACEIs)						
captopril (Capoten)	25 mg (2x daily)	122	27	10		
enalapril (Vasotec)	10 mg	100	17	10	300	282
lisinopril (Prinivil)	10 mg	93	33		134	127
quinapril (Accupril)	10 mg	114	51		200	180

(continued)

Table 16.4   Continued

Drug class	Dose	Cost ($): Generic			Cost ($): Brand name	
Diuretics		Retail	Drugstore .com	Walmart	Retail	Drugstore .com
Angiotensin receptor blockers (ARBs)						
losartan (Cozaar)	50 mg	212	177		270	234
valsartan (Diovan)	160 mg		Coming soon		325	287
irbesartan (Avapro)	150 mg		Coming soon		293	248
Direct renin inhibitor						
aliskiren (Tekturna)	300 mg				387	350
Beta-blockers						
metoprolol succinate (Toprol)	50 mg	94	87		122	110
metoprolol tartrate (Lopressor)	50 mg (2x daily)	102	27	10	369	328
atenolol (Tenormin)	25 mg	77	15	10	173	159
carvedilol (Coreg)	25 mg (2x daily)	400	90	10	494	459
betaxolol (Kerlone)	10 mg	114			146	135
nebivolol (Bystolic)	10 mg				214	198
Alpha-blockers						
doxazosin (Cardura)	1 mg	86	44		174	160

Table 16.5 Sampling of combination drugs: price for a ninety-day supply

Drug class	Dose	Cost as separate drugs:			Cost as combination pills:	
		Generic	Brand	Walmart	Generic	Brand (drugstore.com)
Diuretic/diuretic						
spironolactone/HCTZ	25/25	43		20	47	97
ACEI/diuretic						
enalapril/HCTZ (Vaseretic)	10/25	104		10	73	297
lisinopril/HCTZ (Zestoretic)	20/25	60		10	60	164
quinapril/HCTZ (Accuretic)	20/25	87			87	192
ARB/diuretic						
losartan/HCTZ (Hyzaar)	100/25				269	
olmesartan/HCTZ (Benicar HCT)	40/25		385			361
ACEI/CCB						
benazepril/amlodipine (Lotrel)	20/10				260	462
ARB/CCB						
valsartan/amlodipine (Exforge)	160/10		311			360
ARB/CCB/diuretic						
valsartan/amlodipine/HCTZ (Exforge HCT)			324			310

Table 16.6 Walmart bargains: thirty-day supply: $4; ninety-day supply: $10!

Diuretics	Angiotensin-converting enzyme inhibitors (ACEIs)	Beta-blockers
hydrochlorothiazide	benazepril	atenolol
indapamide	captopril	carvedilol
bumetanide	enalapril	metoprolol tartrate
furosemide	enalapril/hydrochlorothiazide	nadolol
spironolactone	lisinopril	propranolol
triamterene/hydrochlorothiazide	lisinopril/hydrochlorothiazide	
amiloride/hydrochlorothiazide		
	Angiotensin receptor blockers (ARBs)	**Alpha-blockers**
Calcium channel blockers (CCBs)	None at this time	doxazosin
diltiazem (short-acting)		prazosin
verapamil (short-acting)		terazosin
	Vasodilators	**Combination pills**
Central alpha-agonists	hydralazine	atenolol/chlorthalidone
clonidine		bisoprolol/hydrochlorothiazide
guanfacine		
methyldopa		

Anyway, there are many things you can do without resorting to the Canada option (table 16.7).

Generic Medications

Go generic where possible. Walmart $4 plans and online plans offer considerable savings for generic drugs. Although one can argue that a generic version of a drug might not be the true equivalent of the brand name drug, I can't say I've noticed any obvious change in patients' blood pressure when they are switched to a generic drug, and the cost saving is huge.

Occasionally, a patient does report a change in blood pressure, or a side effect, and it is certainly conceivable that the change results from the generic drug being absorbed or metabolized slightly differently than the original drug. More likely though the change can be linked to alterations in diet or activity, or some temporary stress.

Different Drugs from the Same Drug Class

A trickier problem arises when you are taking a drug for which there is no generic version and your health care plan demands that you switch to the generic version of a different drug from within the same drug class. This is now a widespread issue, particularly in prescribing ACEIs and ARBs. For example, there is no generic version of irbesartan (Avapro) (though there will be one soon), and your health care plan asks you to switch from Avapro to a generic version of either a different ARB, such as losartan (Cozaar), or an ACEI, such as lisinopril (Zestril, Prinivil). Are there differences from one drug to another within the same drug class?

Table 16.7 Ways to reduce drug costs

1. Monitor your blood pressure at home.
2. Use generic drugs.
3. Make sure you are on the drug or drugs that are right for you.
4. Get off drugs that are doing nothing.
5. Don't take two drugs that target the same mechanism.
6. The diuretics are as effective as any other drug, and much cheaper.
7. If you need a diuretic, you need to be on a diuretic regimen that is enough to do the job.
8. A good diuretic regimen can eliminate the need for one or more other medications.
9. Ask your doctor to prescribe a double-strength pill that can be broken in half.
10. You will need less medication if you reduce your salt intake and watch your diet.

ACEIs and ARBs: For the most part, one ACEI or ARB will lower blood pressure as much as another, so it is okay to switch from one ACEI to another, one ARB to another, an ACEI to an ARB, or an ARB to an ACEI (unless you have a history of adverse reaction, such as a cough, when previously taking an ACEI). However, there are some exceptions: several studies indicate that losartan (Cozaar) is less effective than other ARBs.[1, 2] A new ARB, azilsartan (Edarbi), appears more effective than other ARBs.[3]

Beta-blockers: Here it is different. As I discuss in chapter 6, the beta-blockers differ from one another much more substantially than most physicians realize. If I select a specific beta-blocker, I usually don't wish to substitute a different one. I discuss at length the advantages and disadvantages of the various beta-blockers in chapter 6.

The Importance of Your Doctor Selecting the Drug That Is Right for You

As I state and restate throughout the book, different patients need different medications. The right drug will control your hypertension; the wrong one won't. If you were started on the wrong drug and it did nothing and your doctor added other drugs that worked, you might be able to come off the first drug. Ask your doctor if that is an option.

If you are on three medications and your blood pressure is still high, your doctor might be able to replace a drug that didn't help with a new one that might, instead of just adding a fourth drug. Also, if you are on three drugs and your hypertension is not under control, I would suggest consulting a hypertension specialist who can steer you onto the medications that are right for you.

Monitor Your Blood Pressure at Home

If your blood pressure is elevated in the doctor's office but is normal at home, you might not need some or all of the medication you are taking. Somewhere between 10 and 20 percent of patients fall into this category; I strongly recommend monitoring your blood pressure at home to find out what your blood pressure is outside the doctor's office.

Don't Take Two Drugs That Target the Same Mechanism

An ACEI and an ARB each targets the RAS. Adding one to the other lowers blood pressure very little. In the ONTARGET trial, this combination lowered blood pressure only 2 millimeters more than either the ACEI (ramipril [Altace]) or the ARB (telmisartan [Micardis]) did by itself.[4] Similarly, adding a DRI (aliskiren [Tekturna]) to an ACEI or ARB will lower blood pressure much less than adding a drug, such as a diuretic, that targets a different mechanism.[5]

The Value of Diuretics

Many patients view a diuretic as "just a water pill" and not as a "pressure pill." Truth is the diuretics lower blood pressure on average just as much as the newest drugs do, and at a fraction of the cost. And in some people, **the blood pressure will never be controlled without the right dose of a diuretic, no matter how many other medications they are taking**. If you are on a few medications but no diuretic, ask your doctor if there is any reason why not.

Increasing the strength of an inexpensive diuretic, or adding a potassium-sparing diuretic (chapter 3), might not only enable you to reduce or stop some of your other medications but might also be the only way your blood pressure can be brought under control. The average diuretic dose is enough for most; but some patients need higher doses, and in many cases their doctors never prescribe them.

Other Options

Another easy strategy: ask your doctor to prescribe pills that are double the dosage you need and break them in half. Thirty pills will last sixty days. You can obtain a pill cutter from your pharmacy.

Finally, lifestyle measures can without doubt reduce your need for medication. Reducing your salt intake might lower your blood pressure as much as 5 or 10 mm or more and reduce the amount of medication you need. A healthy diet will also reduce your need for medication, as will weight loss.

Putting it all together, the advice in this chapter can reduce your drug costs substantially. I cannot emphasize enough the importance of eliminating unnecessary medication, not just because it will save you money, but because it is bad medicine for you to remain on medications that are doing nothing for you and that you don't need.

⓱

CONCLUSION

There is no doubt that millions of people who are being treated for hypertension are on the wrong drugs, doses, and/or combinations. The consequences are not trivial: uncontrolled hypertension, avoidable side effects, excessive medication, and extra costs.

We are fortunate to have many good medications on the market, and with them, hypertension should now be controllable in almost all individuals who take their medication. However, ineffectiveness and side effects are more likely when they are not prescribed correctly.

Patients regularly ask me if any breakthrough medications are on the horizon. The answer, to put it bluntly, is no. With so many effective drugs on the market, it makes little sense for the pharmaceutical industry to invest a fortune looking for new drugs. We will have to do our best with what we have now. Ironically, there are some terrific older drugs that are largely forgotten because of the drug industry's emphasis on, and promotion of, the newer drugs. In essence, old drugs can serve as new drugs for the many physicians who haven't been prescribing them.

Also, the hope that genetic testing could enable us to select the right medication by identifying the genetic defects causing an individual's hypertension will not be fulfilled anytime soon; because there are so many hypertension-related genes, no single gene will be found to have a dominant role in the usual case of hypertension.

The standard guidelines leave enormous gaps when it comes to management of the individual patient. The evidence-based medicine that the guidelines are based on focuses too often on the average response to a drug rather than on how different individuals respond. That is why, despite the many good drugs we have and the many large studies that have been performed, we often get it wrong when we treat the individual patient.

The large studies are not wrong, but they don't address the questions that arise every day in treating individual patients. Worse, hypertension specialists cannot even agree on what the megastudies are telling us and on how their findings are to be translated into clinical practice. Well-designed studies are invaluable in enabling us to discard ineffective treatments and to identify superior ones. But when one treatment is only slightly superior, **choice of treatment should depend more on differences between patients than on the statistically significant but small differences between treatments.**

Evidence-based medicine is largely a good thing. But the studies that it relies on are geared at macrodecisions—decisions pertinent to a large population—and not microdecisions—decisions more pertinent to the individual patient. The approaches I have offered are aimed at the microdecisions—they are about the individual patient, about you.

The truly wonderful news is that we already have many effective medications, and if we use them better, we can bring hypertension under control in almost every case, while reducing side effects, number of medications, and costs. In an era when medical costs are out of control, we can actually spend less and do better by prescribing the right medications. But to do this, we need to be more aware of the clinical clues that can help us in picking and choosing among the drugs.

Ironically, we have a problem of riches. It is often difficult to choose the right drug because there are so many drugs to choose from. When a football coach provides a playbook that has too many plays, his team will usually do better if it focuses on fewer plays but runs them better.

In exactly the same way, the drug treatment of hypertension has become too complicated. Yes, we need a menu of drugs to choose from in different situations. And, yes, we need a few trick plays to use when the going is rough. But we need a playbook that is better organized. It needs to be simplified, so that it is teachable and understandable yet takes into account that different people need different medications. That has not happened.

I have offered a blueprint for selecting drugs. It focuses on matching the drug to the mechanism causing your hypertension. I have emphasized the need to narrow down the number of choices. A physician will have trouble choosing among eight options and will do much better if there are only two or three options that will work in most patients, even if not in all. And when it doesn't work, that is the time to refer to a specialist. Yes, for the sake of the patient, pass the buck.

I am glad I did not write this book twenty years ago, as I have learned much since then, from studies and from clinical experience. And I am certain that I will need to tweak some of my recommendations in the future. Nevertheless, I strongly believe that the core of the approach I have presented to you, taken from scientific knowledge, clinical experience, and critical and logical thinking, is solid and can substantially improve the drug treatment of hypertension for many readers. Also, given the likelihood that we will have no new drugs and no new treatment-related insights from genetic studies in the next several years, I believe my recommendations will hold true for many years to come.

I hope the book will help you in getting on to the medication that is right for you. I cannot emphasize enough though that you should not make any medication changes on your own. There might be factors that dictate why your doctor chose medication A and not medication B. By raising the question with your doctor, he can communicate why he chose a certain medication or why he prefers not to prescribe a different one. He might also agree that it is reasonable to try a different medication, cut one out, or change the dose of another.

If your blood pressure is controlled and you feel well, there may be no need to change your medication. But if your blood pressure is not under control, if you are experiencing side effects, or if you are on more medications than you think you should need, it would be important to consider changes. And if your doctor does not wish to change your medication, she owes you an explanation as to why not. Your reasonable question merits a reasonable answer.

Finally, I cannot overstate the importance of diet and exercise in managing your hypertension. If you really want to reduce medication, and its associated costs and side effects, the best and healthiest way is to reduce your sodium intake (if you have salt-sensitive hypertension [chapter 10]), lose weight, and exercise. **With diet and exercise, I believe that half of all the medication prescribed for hypertension could be eliminated.** You may still need medication but less.

With the increase in obesity and decrease in fitness in our country and with the survival of most people to old age, we are assured of an epidemic of

hypertension for a long time to come. In the past thirty years, one drug after another has come onto the market and radically improved our ability to
control hypertension. However, we can no longer expect to see new drugs
come along. The good news, however, is that we already have enough effective drugs to control hypertension in almost all cases, and usually without
side effects. It is wrong to believe that your hypertension is uncontrollable
or that you have to live with side effects the rest of your life, except in the
unusual case.

Newer invasive procedures, such as interruption of the sympathetic
nerves to the kidney, hold promise in lowering blood pressure in patients
with truly uncontrollable hypertension. But I strongly believe that it will be
the rare patient in whom there will be a need to resort to such procedures

The good news also is that you won't develop "immunity" or resistance to
the blood pressure drugs that have lowered your blood pressure. We don't
develop resistance to antihypertensive drugs the way we do to the effect of
antibiotics. You can expect the drug you are taking to continue to work for
decades, although the medication may need to be tweaked as we get older
or fatter, or if other factors enter the picture.

Finally, the good news is that hypertension need not shorten or impair
your life. With the drugs we have today, almost everyone with hypertension
can expect to achieve a normal blood pressure and reduced cardiovascular
risk, while feeling well and living a full and long life. The key is an interested physician and, more important, an interested patient.

NOTES

Introduction

1. Vital signs: prevalence, treatment, and control of hypertension—United States, 1999–2002 and 2005–2008. *MMWR Morb Mortal Wkly Rep* 2011;60:103–8.

Chapter 1

1. Mancia G, Facchetti R, Bombelli M, et al. Long-term risk of mortality associated with selective and combined elevation in office, home, and ambulatory blood pressure. *Hypertension* 2006;47:846–53.

2. Pickering TG, Hall JE, Appel LJ, et al. Recommendations for blood pressure measurement in humans and experimental animals: Part 1: Blood pressure measurement in humans: a statement for professionals from the Subcommittee of Professional and Public Education of the American Heart Association Council on High Blood Pressure Research. *Hypertension* 2005;45:142–61.

3. Ugajin T, Hozawa A, Ohkubo T, et al. White-coat hypertension as a risk factor for the development of home hypertension: the Ohasama study. *Arch Intern Med* 2005;165:1541–6.

4. Cohen DL, Townsend RR. Masked hypertension: an increasingly common but often unrecognized issue in hypertension management. *J Clin Hypertens* 2010;12:522–3.

5. Parati G, Stergiou GS, Asmar R, et al. European Society of Hypertension practice guidelines for home blood pressure monitoring. *J Hum Hypertens* 2010;24:779–85.

6. Palatini P, Ceolotto G, Ragazzo F, et al. CYP1A2 genotype modifies the association between coffee intake and the risk of hypertension. *J Hypertens* 2009;27:1594–601.

7. Mann SJ. Systolic hypertension in the elderly. Pathophysiology and management. *Arch Intern Med* 1992;152:1977–84.

8. Kannel WB. Hypertension and other risk factors in coronary heart disease. *Am Heart J* 1987;114:918–25.

9. Beckett NS, Peters R, Fletcher AE, et al. Treatment of hypertension in patients 80 years of age or older. *N Engl J Med* 2008;358:1887–98.

10. Mann SJ. Job stress and blood pressure: a critical appraisal of reported studies. *Curr Hypertens Rev* 2006;2:127–38.

Chapter 3

1. Messerli FH, Makani H, Benjo A, et al. Antihypertensive efficacy of hydrochlorothiazide as evaluated by ambulatory blood pressure monitoring: a meta-analysis of randomized trials. *J Am Coll Cardiol* 2011;57:590–600.

2. Dorsch MP, Gillespie BW, Erickson SR, et al. Chlorthalidone reduces cardiovascular events compared with hydrochlorothiazide: a retrospective cohort analysis. *Hypertension* 2011;57:689–94.

3. Baumgart P. Torasemide in comparison with thiazides in the treatment of hypertension. *Cardiovasc Drugs Ther* 1993;7:63–8.

Chapter 4

1. Dickerson JE, Hingorani AD, Ashby MJ, et al. Optimisation of antihypertensive treatment by crossover rotation of four major classes. *Lancet* 1999;353:2008–13.

2. Kiowski W, Bühler FR, Fadayomi MO. Age, race, blood pressure and renin: predictors for antihypertensive treatment with calcium antagonists. *Am J Cardiol* 1986;56:81H–5H.

3. Cappuccio FP, Markandu ND, Singer DR, et al. A double-blind crossover study of the effect of concomitant diuretic therapy in hypertensive patients treated with amlodipine. *Am J Hypertens* 1991;4:297–302.

Chapter 5

1. Kassler-Taub K, Littlejohn T, Elliott W, et al. Comparative efficacy of two angiotensin II receptor antagonists, irbesartan and losartan in mild-to-moderate hypertension. Irbesartan/Losartan Study Investigators. *Am J Hypertens* 1998;11:445–53.

2. Smith DH, Dubiel R, Jones M. Use of 24-hour ambulatory blood pressure monitoring to assess antihypertensive efficacy: a comparison of olmesartan medoxomil, losartan potassium, valsartan, and irbesartan. *Am J Cardiovasc Drugs* 2005;5:41–50.

3. White WB, Weber MA, Sica D, et al. Effects of the angiotensin receptor blocker azilsartan medoxomil versus olmesartan and valsartan on ambulatory and clinic blood pressure in patients with stages 1 and 2 hypertension. *Hypertension* 2011;57:413–20.

4. Yusuf S, Teo KK, Pogue J, et al. Telmisartan, ramipril, or both in patients at high risk for vascular events. *N Engl J Med* 2008;358:1547–59.

5. Sipahi I, Debanne SM, Rowland DY, et al. Angiotensin-receptor blockade and risk of cancer: meta-analysis of randomised controlled trials. *Lancet Oncol* 2010;11:627–36.

6. Bangalore S, Kumar S, Kjeldsen SE, et al. Antihypertensive drugs and risk of cancer: network meta-analyses and trial sequential analyses of 324,168 participants from randomised trials. *Lancet Oncol* 2011;12:65–82.

7. Oparil S, Yarows SA, Patel S, et al. Dual inhibition of the renin system by aliskiren and valsartan. *Lancet* 2007;370:1126–7.

8. Dahlöf B, Devereux RB, Kjeldsen SE, et al. Cardiovascular morbidity and mortality in the Losartan Intervention For Endpoint reduction in hypertension study (LIFE): a randomised trial against atenolol. *Lancet* 2002;359:995–1003.

Chapter 6

1. Dahlöf B, Devereux RB, Kjeldsen SE, et al. Cardiovascular morbidity and mortality in the Losartan Intervention For Endpoint reduction in hypertension study (LIFE): a randomised trial against atenolol. *Lancet* 2002;359:995–1003.

2. Bakris GL, Fonseca V, Katholi RE, et al. Metabolic effects of carvedilol vs metoprolol in patients with type 2 diabetes mellitus and hypertension: a randomized controlled trial. *JAMA* 2004;292:2227–36.

3. Mann SJ. Neurogenic essential hypertension revisited: the case for increased clinical and research attention. *Am J Hypertens* 2003;16:881–8.

4. Ko DT, Hebert PR, Coffey CS, et al. Beta-blocker therapy and symptoms of depression, fatigue, and sexual dysfunction. *JAMA* 2002;288:351–7.

5. Sharma AM, Pischon T, Hardt S, et al. Hypothesis: Beta-adrenergic receptor blockers and weight gain: a systematic analysis. *Hypertension* 2001;37:250–4.

Chapter 7

1. Major cardiovascular events in hypertensive patients randomized to doxazosin vs chlorthalidone: the antihypertensive and lipid-lowering treatment to prevent heart attack trial (ALLHAT). ALLHAT Collaborative Research Group. *JAMA* 2000;283:1967–75.

2. Mann SJ, Gerber LM. Low-dose alpha/beta blockade in the treatment of essential hypertension. *Am J Hypertens* 2001;14:553–8.

3. Torp-Pedersen C, Poole-Wilson PA, Swedberg K, et al. Effects of metoprolol and carvedilol on cause-specific mortality and morbidity in patients with chronic heart failure–COMET. *Amer Heart J* 2005;149:370–6.

4. Mann SJ. Neurogenic essential hypertension revisited: the case for increased clinical and research attention. *Am J Hypertens* 2003;16:881–8.

5. Mann SJ. Drug therapy for resistant hypertension: simplifying the approach. *J Clin Hypertens* 2011;13:120–30.

6. Mann SJ, Gerber LM. Low-dose alpha/beta blockade in the treatment of essential hypertension. *Am J Hypertens* 2001;14:553–8.

7. Searle M, Dathan R, Dean S, et al. Doxazosin in combination with atenolol in essential hypertension: a double-blind placebo-controlled multicentre trial. *Eur J Clin Pharmacol* 1990;39:299–300.

8. Holtzman JL, Kaihlanen PM, Rider JA, et al. Concomitant administration of terazosin and atenolol for the treatment of essential hypertension. *Arch Intern Med* 1988;148:539–43.

9. Morgan T. Clinical pharmacokinetics and pharmacodynamics of carvedilol. *Clin Pharmacokinet* 1994;26:335–46.

10. Prichard BN, Richards DA. Comparison of labetalol with other anti-hypertensive drugs. *Br J Clin Pharmacol* 1982;13:41S–7S.

Chapter 9

1. Materson BJ, Reda DJ, Cushman WC, et al. Single-drug therapy for hypertension in men. A comparison of six antihypertensive agents with placebo. The Department of Veterans Affairs Cooperative Study Group on Antihypertensive Agents. *N Engl J Med* 1993;328:914–21.

2. Jamerson K, Weber MA, Bakris GL, et al. Benazepril plus amlodipine or hydrochlorothiazide for hypertension in high-risk patients. *N Engl J Med* 2008;359:2417–28.

3. Brown MJ. Hypertension and ethnic group. *BMJ* 2006;332:833–6.

Chapter 10

1. Mann SJ. Drug therapy for resistant hypertension: simplifying the approach. *J Clin Hypertens* 2011;13:120–30.

2. Mann SJ, Parikh NS. A simplified mechanistic algorithm for treating resistant hypertension: efficacy in a retrospective study. *J Clin Hypertens* 2012 (in press).

3. Pimenta E, Gaddam KK, Oparil S, et al. Effects of dietary sodium reduction on blood pressure in subjects with resistant hypertension: results from a randomized trial. *Hypertension* 2009;54:475–81.

4. Setaro JF, Black HR. Refractory hypertension. *N Engl J Med* 1992;327:543–7.

5. Garg JP, Elliott WJ, Folker A, et al. Resistant hypertension revisited: a comparison of two university-based cohorts. *Am J Hypertens* 2005;18:619–26.

Chapter 11

1. Mann SJ. *Healing Hypertension: A Revolutionary New Approach* (New York: Wiley, 1999).

2. Jorgensen RS, Johnson BT, Kolodziej ME, et al. Elevated blood pressure and personality: a meta-analytic review. *Psychol Bull* 1996;120:293–320.

3. Suls J, Wan CK, Costa Jr PT. Relationship of trait anger to resting blood pressure: a meta-analysis. *Health Psychol* 1995;14:444–56.

4. Mann SJ, James GD. Defensiveness and essential hypertension. *J Psychosom Res* 1998;45:139–48.

5. Mann SJ. Job stress and blood pressure: a critical appraisal of reported studies. *Curr Hypertens Rev* 2006;2:127–38.

6. Eisenberg DM, Delbanco TL, Berkey CS, et al. Cognitive behavioral techniques for hypertension: are they effective? *Ann Intern Med* 1993;118:964–72.

7. MacMillan HL, Fleming JE, Trocmé N, et al. Prevalence of child physical and sexual abuse in the community. Results from the Ontario Health Supplement. *JAMA* 1997;278:131–5.

8. Mann SJ. Severe paroxysmal hypertension (pseudopheochromocytoma): understanding the cause and treatment. *Arch Intern Med* 1999;159:670–4.

9. Mann SJ. Severe paroxysmal hypertension (pseudopheochromocytoma). *Curr Hypertens Rep* 2008;10:12–8.

10. Mann SJ. Neurogenic essential hypertension revisited: the case for increased clinical and research attention. *Am J Hypertens* 2003;16:881–8.

11. Julius S. The blood pressure seeking properties of the central nervous system. *J Hypertens* 1988;6:177–85.

12. Mann SJ, Gerber LM. Psychological characteristics and responses to antihypertensive drug therapy. *J Clin Hypertens* 2002;4:25–34.

Chapter 12

1. Epstein M, Calhoun DA. The role of aldosterone in resistant hypertension: implications for pathogenesis and therapy. *Curr Hypertens Rep* 2007;9:98–105.

2. Mann SJ, Sos TA. Misleading results of randomized trials: the example of renal artery stenting. *J Clin Hypertens* 2010;12:1–2.

Chapter 13

1. Cheung BM, Ong KL, Man YB, et al. Prevalence, awareness, treatment, and control of hypertension: United States National Health and Nutrition Examination Survey 2001–2002. *J Clin Hypertens* 2006;8:93–8.

2. Beckett NS, Peters R, Fletcher AE, et al. Treatment of hypertension in patients 80 years of age or older. *N Engl J Med* 2008;358:1887–98.

3. Materson BJ, Reda DJ, Cushman WC, et al. Single-drug therapy for hypertension in men. A comparison of six antihypertensive agents with placebo. The Department of Veterans Affairs Cooperative Study Group on Antihypertensive Agents. *N Engl J Med* 1993;328:914–21.

4. Prevention of stroke by antihypertensive drug treatment in older persons with isolated systolic hypertension. Final results of the Systolic Hypertension in the Elderly Program (SHEP). SHEP Cooperative Research Group. *JAMA* 1991;265:3255–64.

5. Staessen JA, Thijs L, Fagard RH, et al. Calcium channel blockade and cardiovascular prognosis in the European trial on isolated systolic hypertension. *Hypertension* 1998;32:410–6.

Chapter 14

1. Radack K, Deck CC. Are oral decongestants safe in hypertension? An evaluation of the evidence and a framework for assessing clinical trials. *Ann Allergy* 1986;56:396–401.

2. Pope JE, Anderson JJ, Felson DT. A meta-analysis of the effects of nonsteroidal anti-inflammatory drugs on blood pressure. *Arch Intern Med* 1993;153:477–84.

3. Snowden S, Nelson R. The effects of nonsteroidal anti-inflammatory drugs on blood pressure in hypertensive patients. *Cardiol Rev* 2011;19:184–91.

4. McGettigan P, Henry D. Cardiovascular risk and inhibition of cyclooxygenase: a systematic review of the observational studies of selective and nonselective inhibitors of cyclooxygenase 2. *JAMA* 2006;296:1633–44.

5. Mann SJ, Pickering TG, Alderman MH, et al. Assessment of the effects of alpha- and beta-blockade in hypertensive patients who smoke cigarettes. *Am J Med* 1989;86:79–81.

6. Palatini P, Ceolotto G, Ragazzo F, et al. CYP1A2 genotype modifies the association between coffee intake and the risk of hypertension. *J Hypertens* 2009;27:1594–601.

Chapter 15

1. Wiley RL, Dunn CL, Cox RH, et al. Isometric exercise training lowers resting blood pressure. *Med Sci Sports Exerc* 1992;24:749–54.

Chapter 16

1. Smith DH, Dubiel R, Jones M. Use of 24-hour ambulatory blood pressure monitoring to assess antihypertensive efficacy: a comparison of olmesartan medoxomil, losartan potassium, valsartan, and irbesartan. *Am J Cardiovasc Drugs* 2005;5:41–50.

2. Kassler-Taub K, Littlejohn T, Elliott W, et al. Comparative efficacy of two angiotensin II receptor antagonists, irbesartan and losartan in mild-to-moderate hypertension. Irbesartan/Losartan Study Investigators. *Am J Hypertens* 1998;11:445–53.

3. White WB, Weber MA, Sica D, et al. Effects of the angiotensin receptor blocker azilsartan medoxomil versus olmesartan and valsartan on ambulatory and clinic blood pressure in patients with stages 1 and 2 hypertension. *Hypertension* 2011;57:413–20.

4. Yusuf S, Teo KK, Pogue J, et al. Telmisartan, ramipril, or both in patients at high risk for vascular events. *N Engl J Med* 2008;358:1547–59.

5. Oparil S, Yarows SA, Patel S, et al. Dual inhibition of the renin system by aliskiren and valsartan. *Lancet* 2007;370:1126–7.

INDEX

ABOUT THE AUTHOR

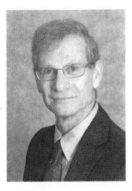

Dr. Samuel J. Mann is one of a relatively small number of physicians who specialize specifically in the treatment of hypertension. He is a professor of clinical medicine at the Hypertension Center of the New York Presbyterian Hospital–Weill Cornell Medical Center, where he has a large consultation practice and is involved in hypertension research. He is the author of fifty scientific articles, a dozen book chapters, and a book, *Healing Hypertension: A Revolutionary New Approach* (1999). His recent research has focused on the management of hard-to-control hypertension, and on the role of the mind/body connection in understanding and treating hypertension.

In *Hypertension and You*, he focuses on what is wrong with how blood pressure medications are prescribed, and provides information and strategies that are not found in previous books. He explains how we can do much better in controlling hypertension and reducing the risk of stroke and heart attack, while reducing medication, side effects and costs, by using the right medications in the right patients.

CPSIA information can be obtained at www.ICGtesting.com
Printed in the USA
BVOW082219070313

315009BV00002B/3/P